RAY/08.

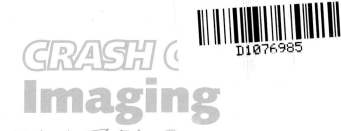

CRASH C

Imaging

616.0754. BiC

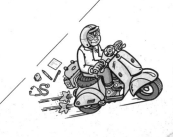

Dedication
For Susan, Katie & Rosie BEK
Mum, Dad & Haiza ICB

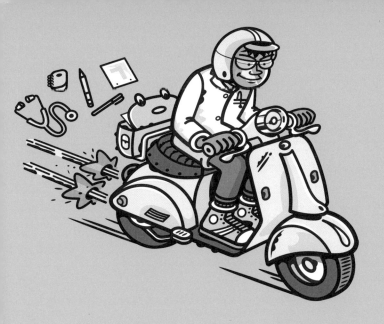

Series editor
Daniel Horton-Szar
BSc (Hons) MB BS (Hons) MRCGP
Northgate Medical Practice
Canterbury
Kent

with contributions by

Nigel Wethers
Superintendent Radiographer,
Royal Victoria Hospital, The
Queen's University, Belfast, UK

Peter Flynn
Consultant Neuroradiologist,
Royal Victoria Hospital, The
Queen's University, Belfast, UK

Annie Paterson
Consultant Paediatric Radiologist,
Royal Belfast Hospital for Sick
Children, Belfast, UK

Imaging

Barry Kelly MD FRCS(Ed) FRCR FFRRCSI
Consultant Radiologist, The Royal Victoria Hospital; Honorary Senior Lecturer in Radiology,
The Queen's University, Belfast, UK

Ian C Bickle MB BCh BAO(Hons)
Specialist Registrar in Radiology, North Trent Training Scheme, Royal Hallamshire Hospital,
Sheffield, UK

ELSEVIER
MOSBY

Edinburgh • London • New York • Oxford • Philadelphia • St Louis
Sydney • Toronto 2007

ELSEVIER
MOSBY

MOSBY
An imprint of Elsevier Limited

Commissioning Editor	**Fiona Conn**
Development Editor	**Ailsa Laing**
Project Manager	**Frances Affleck**
Designer	**Andy Chapman**
Illustrator	**Amanda Walker**

First published 2007

ISBN-13   978-0-7234-3192-3
ISBN-10   0-7234-3192-2

British Library Cataloguing in Publication Data
A catalogue record for this book is available from the British Library

Library of Congress Cataloging in Publication Data
A catalog record for this book is available from the Library of Congress

---

Notice

Neither the Publisher nor the Authors assume any responsibility for any loss or injury and/or damage to persons or property arising out of or related to any use of the material contained in this book. It is the responsibility of the treating practitioner, relying on independent expertise and knowledge of the patient, to determine the best treatment and method of application for the patient.

The Publisher

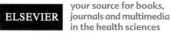

your source for books,
journals and multimedia
in the health sciences
www.elsevierhealth.com

The
Publisher's
policy is to use
**paper manufactured
from sustainable forests**

Printed in Italy

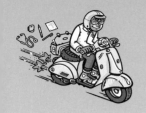

Author Preface

Medical imaging plays an increasingly integral part of the day-to-day management of patients. With continued diagnostic advances in both cross-sectional diagnostic and therapeutic interventional modalities, the place of radiology has never been more central in patient management. For this reason it is essential that all junior doctors have a grasp of basic radiology.

Modern medicine presents a bewildering array of facts, tests, procedures and diagnoses for the beginner. Selecting the most appropriate imaging investigations for your patient is one of these challenges.

In this book, we have used the popular format of the 'Crash Course' series, to instruct those taking their first tentative steps into the world of clinical imaging. The book is focused and instructive, but not exhaustive. We have attempted to guide the reader from the starting point of a clinical complaint, e.g. shortness of breath or altered bowel habit. An algorithm for investigating the symptom and potential imaging findings is described and evaluated. This is accompanied by a gallery of images of core diseases in each body system. *Crash Course: Imaging* will also provide the understanding and skills to approach the key X-ray images which now feature regularly in OSCE-based final examinations.

A wise academic once said, 'For every mistake made from lack of knowledge, ten are made from lack of looking'.

It is our hope that this book will show the reader how to look, and provide the background information, to consolidate their knowledge base.

BEK
ICB
Belfast and Sheffield

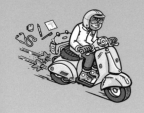

Series Preface

More than a decade has now passed since work began on the first titles of the *Crash Course* series, but medicine never stands still and the work of keeping this series relevant for today's students is an ongoing process. This title builds upon the success of the preceding books, keeping the series up to date with the latest medical research and developments in pharmacology and current best practice.

As always, we listen to feedback from the thousands of students who use *Crash Course* and have made further improvements to the layout and structure of the books. We have also worked to integrate points of clinical relevance into the basic medical science material, which will not only add to the interest of the text but will reinforce the principles being described.

Despite fully revising the books, we hold fast to the principles on which we first developed the series: *Crash Course* will always bring you all the information you need to revise in compact, manageable volumes that integrate basic medical science and clinical practice. The books still maintain the balance between clarity and conciseness, and providing sufficient depth for those aiming at distinction. The authors are medical students and junior doctors who have recent experience of the exams you are now facing, and the accuracy of the material is checked by senior faculty members from across the UK.

I wish you all the best for your future careers!

Dr Dan Horton-Szar
Series Editor

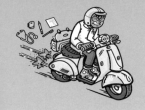

Contents

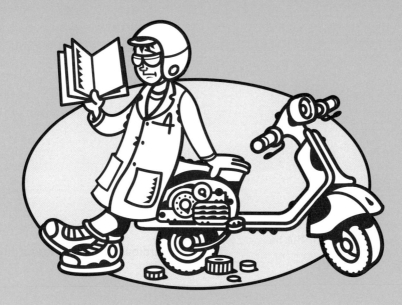

THE PATIENT PRESENTS WITH

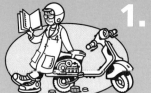

1. Chest Pain, Dyspnoea or Haemoptysis

Chest pain, dyspnoea and haemoptysis are frequent reasons for medical admission. With the large prevalence of ischaemic heart disease in the western world, acute coronary syndromes should always be at the forefront of the clinician's mind. As the vast majority of chest pain arises from either cardiovascular or respiratory pathology, the plain chest radiograph (CXR) is the usual first-line imaging step.

 Haemoptysis in a smoker over 50 years of age is caused by bronchogenic carcinoma until proven otherwise.

The finding of a normal CXR does not exclude significant pathology. This is particularly the case with pulmonary embolic (PE) disease, the chest radiograph often being unremarkable. Here, the focus moves to appropriate further imaging—either to look for disease not identified on CXR, but for which there is a high clinical suspicion, or to further evaluate an equivocal area of abnormality on plain film. Clearly, particular attention should be paid to excluding an acute cause that would warrant urgent attention, e.g. pneumothorax, dissecting aneurysm or pericardial tamponade.

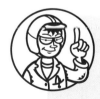 Request an expiratory film if a pneumothorax is suspected. In expiration there is relatively increased intrapleural pressure and the lung edge is maximally displaced from the chest wall.

In many instances, CT of the chest would be the next imaging step—the widened mediastinum on a trauma patient's CXR suggesting aortic dissection; the cavitating mass in the right middle lobe, a bronchogenic carcinoma.

 Squamous cell carcinoma is the commonest bronchogenic carcinoma to cavitate.

A VQ scan is more appropriate if the clinical suspicion is of a PE and the CXR is normal. CT pulmonary angiography should be performed if the CXR is abnormal. Although infrequently undertaken by the radiologist, remember the important role of echocardiography and coronary angiography in cardiovascular pathologies—a vital tool in imaging cardiac and pericardial disease.

Cardiovascular disorders

Ischaemic heart disease
The chest x-ray is usually normal. However, pacemakers and prosthetic valves are frequent findings. Sternotomy wires and graft clips may be identified. It is also possible to see calcification of the aorta or the left ventricle. This latter feature is usually related to a left ventricular aneurysm.

 The diameter of a prosthetic heart valve is inversely proportional to the pressure across it.

Left ventricular failure (see Fig. 20.5)
Chest x-ray features (Fig. 1.1) include (as disease progresses):
- Cardiomegaly (cardiothoracic ratio >0.5).
- Increased vascularity to the upper zones and decreased vascularity to the bases.
- Discrete vessels seen in the outer third of the lung fields.
- Kerley B lines at the basal lung periphery (interlobular septal thickening).
- Air space consolidation (pulmonary oedema).
- Pleural effusions.

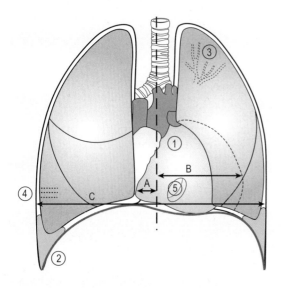

Fig. 1.1 Radiographic features of CCF on CXR: 1. Cardiomegaly (A+B/C = CT ratio >0.50); 2. Pleural effusion; 3. Upper lobe diversion; 4. Kerley B lines; 5. Possible underlying cause (e.g. mitral valve replacement).

Pericarditis

In acute pericarditis, the chest x-ray is often unremarkable, but radiological signs of pericardial effusion (see Fig. 20.12) would include an enlarged globular or 'water bottle' heart. In the chronic form, pericardial calcification can be seen, especially in the atrioventricular groove and the less pulsatile areas. Sparing of the cardiac apex is a recognized feature.

Aortic dissection

The chest x-ray signs can be conveniently divided into those due to the dissection itself and those due to subsequent rupture.

With dissection, there is:
• Widening of the mediastinum.
• Depression of the left main bronchus.
• Contralateral displacement of a nasogastric (NG) tube (if present).

A useful marker is aortic calcification: if present in the arch on the chest radiograph, this defines the intima. Thus the thickness of the arch wall (intima–adventitia) can be calculated. Normally this is less than 6 mm. If there is a dissection, it

will occur between these layers and therefore the arch wall thickness increases and the calcification is displaced towards the lumen. If the arch wall is of normal thickness, and the NG tube and left main bronchus are normally placed, the possibility of dissection becomes very unlikely.

With rupture, there is evidence of blood in the left chest. This is manifested by apical capping and pleural blood. It is important to remember that if the patient is supine when x-rayed, the pleural blood will lie behind the lung and on the CXR that side will be greyer (less dark) than the other side. This is known as 'veiling' of the lung. In addition, the descending aortic shadow, normally visible behind the heart, will be absent as its silhouette will be obscured (effaced) by blood.

In traumatic transections, the dissection classically occurs at the aortic isthmus—that portion of the aorta just distal to the left subclavian artery where the mobile arch joins the fixed descending thoracic aorta.

On CT scans, the aortic dissection is seen as a flap within the lumen (see Fig. 20.8). Blood is identified around the aorta within the mediastinum (Fig. 1.2). The gold standard investigation is angiography which will confirm the dissection as a contour abnormality, with contrast accumulation within the dissection or the flap itself; however, multidetector (multislice) CT is increasingly replacing catheter angiography as the definitive diagnostic imaging test.

Respiratory disorders

Pneumonia

Pneumonia typically manifests itself on the CXR as a region of increased density. This density represents the 'consolidated' acini surrounding the air-filled bronchial tree (the 'air bronchogram'). There are four common types of pneumonia in clinical practice: lobar pneumonia, bronchopneumonia, interstitial pneumonia and cavitating pneumonia.

Lobar pneumonia

Lobar pneumonia affects and therefore delineates a lobe of the lung. The affected lobe can be identified by applying the 'silhouette' sign. This sign indicates that, normally, the heart and

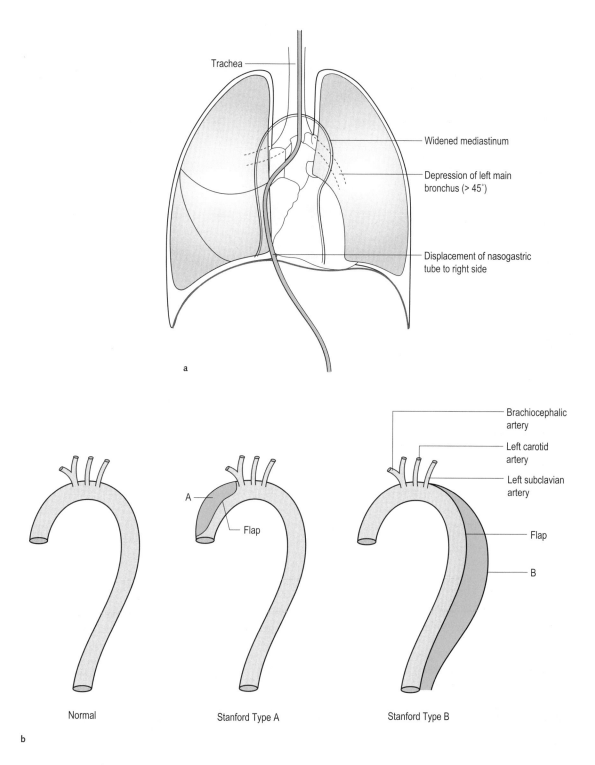

Fig. 1.2 Features of aortic dissection: (a) on CXR; (b) on coronal CT/MR.

diaphragm can be visualized because their silhouettes are surrounded by air in the lungs. If a lobe loses its air (e.g. by being consolidated), then the structure that it abuts cannot be identified and is said to be effaced, i.e. not visible (Figs 1.3, 1.4; see also Figs 19.11, 19.23).

Following consolidation comes collapse. This is diagnosed by volume loss within the lung. Left lower lobe collapse, for example, produces elevation of the hemidiaphragm (Fig. 1.5) and depression (downward displacement) of the hilum. The commonest pathogen is pneumococcus.

Lobar consolidation	
Consolidated lobe	**Structure effaced**
Left upper	Aortic knuckle (Fig. 1.4a)
Lingula	Left heart border (Fig. 1.4a)
Left lower	Left hemidiaphragm (Fig. 1.4b)
Right upper	Right superior mediastinum (Fig. 1.4e)
Right middle	Right heart border (Fig. 1.4d)
Right lower	Right hemidiaphragm (Fig. 1.4c)

Fig. 1.3 Lobar consolidation.

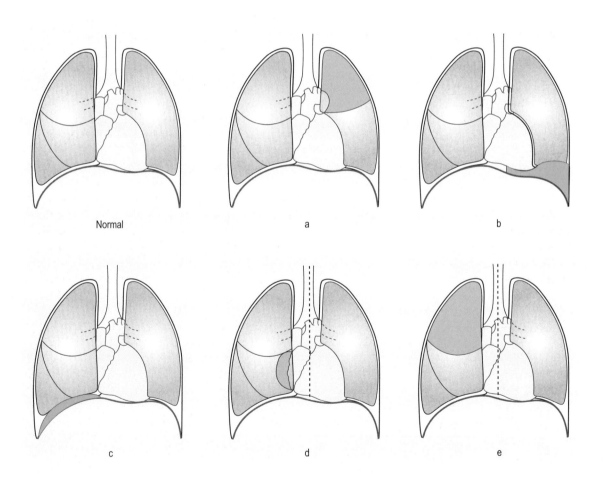

Fig. 1.4 Silhouette signs of consolidation on CXR: (a) left upper lobe (no distinct aortic knuckle); (b) left lower lobe (loss of left hemidiaphragm silhouette); (c) right lower lobe (loss of right hemidiaphragm); (d) right middle lobe (loss of right heart border); (e) right upper lobe (consolidation limited by horizontal fissure).

6

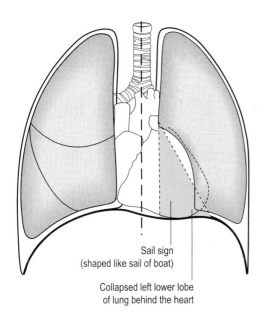

Sail sign
(shaped like sail of boat)

Collapsed left lower lobe
of lung behind the heart

Fig. 1.5 Left lower lobe collapse ('sail' sign).

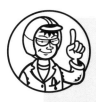 The chest X-ray should be repeated within 4–6 weeks following therapy to ensure that there has been complete resolution of the consolidation.

Bronchopneumonia

The characteristic pattern in bronchopneumonia is multifocal lobular areas of consolidation. These densities are frequently ill defined. 'Spared' or normal lobules between affected areas lead to what has been termed a 'patchwork quilt'. The primary sites of involvement are the terminal and respiratory bronchioles, with disease spreading through the tracheobronchial tree.

Interstitial pneumonia

Interstitial pneumonia usually starts in the bronchus and bronchioles and extends into the interstitium. Interstitial lung disease typically produces widening of the interstitium throughout the lung. These widened structures appear as lines or, when viewed end on, as dots. Therefore, in interstitial pneumonias look for lines and dots throughout the lung. Common causes of interstitial

pneumonia are mycoplasma, chlamydia and viruses, especially influenza, varicella and cytomegalovirus. The commonest two viral pathogens—varicella and influenza—can present with multifocal consolidation. In the latter case, the consolidation is classically perihilar. Immunosuppressed patients, including those with AIDS, are more susceptible (see Fig. 19.12).

Cavitating pneumonia

Cavitation is seen with many pathogens and can be very difficult to distinguish radiologically from carcinoma. Organisms responsible include staphylococcus, tuberculosis and klebsiella. Aspiration and Gram-negative pneumonias can also cause cavitation (see Fig. 19.14).

Pulmonary embolus

The chest x-ray is unreliable in the diagnosis of pulmonary embolus (PE) and its main function is to exclude other causes of the patient's symptomatology. However, there are recognized signs of PE on the chest x-ray, the most common being unilateral hypoperfusion (oligaemia) in one lung. This is called the Westermark sign.

Ventilation perfusion (VQ) imaging demonstrates an embolism by displaying a region which is ventilated (by the open bronchus) but not perfused (as the artery is occluded by thrombus/ embolus). This ventilation–perfusion combination is known as a mismatch. VQ scans are reported as low, intermediate or high probability for PE. The latter two categories usually require treatment. The accuracy of the examination can be undermined by coexistent acute or chronic pulmonary disease. A recent chest radiograph should accompany the patient attending for VQ imaging.

CT scanning

On CT, the embolic material is seen as a black filling defect within the opacified white pulmonary artery (see Fig. 19.20). This is known as the 'polo-mint' sign, seen on axial section. The excellent image resolution of multidetector (multislice) CTs has allowed the diagnosis of pulmonary emboli to be made in smaller segmental arterial branches (Fig. 1.6).

Pneumothorax

The appearances of pneumothorax differ in the erect and the supine chest x-ray (Fig. 1.7). On the erect film, the pneumothorax is seen as a stripe of air between the lung edge and the chest wall (see Fig. 19.13). It is more clearly appreciated on the expiratory film, as the relatively increased intrapleural pressure maximizes the size of the pneumothorax. On a supine film, the free gas lies anterior to the lung so tends to manifest as a deep costophrenic sulcus or as an accentuation of the heart border.

Thoracic malignancy

Primary thoracic malignancy on chest x-ray has a variety of radiological appearances, none of which is specific, but all are generally suspicious; for example, a hilar mass (see Fig. 19.17), particularly if irregular or spiculated; a solitary pulmonary nodule, particularly if cavitated; or an apical mass (see Fig. 19.16) should all arouse suspicion. Some malignancies, particularly bronchoalveolar carcinoma and lymphoma, can appear as areas of non-resolving pneumonia. Further radiological investigation is with CT, which will localize the lesion anatomically and identify lymphadenopathy and pulmonary or bony metastases (see Fig. 19.22b). Magnetic resonance imaging (MRI) is usually reserved for peripheral lesions to exclude chest wall involvement. Positron emission tomography (PET) scanning is proving effective in confirming the nature of the tumour, staging the disease and identifying recurrent disease in glucose-avid lesions (see Part II, Principles of Radiology).

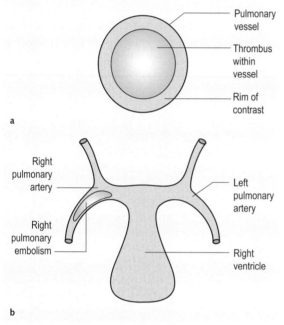

Fig. 1.6 Pulmonary embolus CT: (a) axial with 'polo-mint' sign; (b) longitudinal.

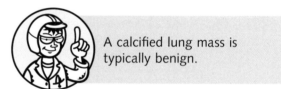

A calcified lung mass is typically benign.

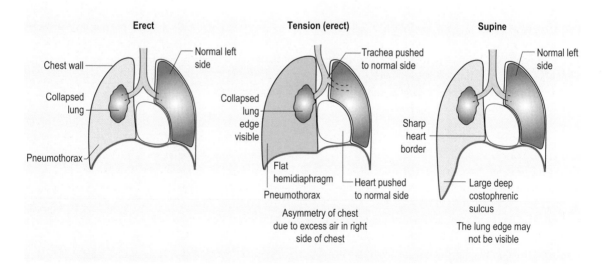

Fig. 1.7 Difference between erect/supine CXR features of pneumothorax.

Metastases

Almost all primary malignancies can metastasize to the lung (see Fig. 19.22a).

Pulmonary metastases are usually seen as multiple circular densities. Common malignancies which metastasize to lung include testicular, renal, thyroid, breast and colon cancer, lymphomas and sarcomas. Some have relatively specific appearances, e.g. thyroid, which can be tiny and multiple ('miliary') metastases, and renal or sarcomatous metastases ('cannonball'). Calcification is associated with osteogenic sarcoma and colloid metastases, e.g. colon.

Case conferences

Case 1

A 75-year-old male patient is admitted with sudden onset chest pain radiating to the back between the shoulder blades. On examination he is hypertensive (195/99) and a 20 mmHg systolic disparity is noted between the right and left arms. His old medical notes outline a 12-year history of hypertension requiring multiple antihypertensive medications.

Chest x-ray

The heart is enlarged. Pulmonary vascularity is normal, but the mediastinum is widened. The descending aortic shadow is absent. There is no active lung lesion. There is no evidence of an apical cap, nor of a pleural effusion.

CT chest and abdomen

A dynamically enhanced helical CT scan has been performed with contrast administered via the left arm (see Fig. 19.15).

There is an abnormality of the aortic arch with a 'flap' seen beginning distal to the left subclavian artery and extending down the descending thoracic aorta to the upper abdomen. Two lumena—the 'true' and the 'false'—are seen and both are opacified with contrast. There is no abnormality seen relating to the pericardium or ascending arch. There is no pleural fluid collection.

Within the abdomen, contrast opacifies both the coeliac and superior mesenteric arteries. Both renal arteries and kidneys are also opacified and, at the level of the renal arteries, the aortic lumen is normal.

Conclusion

The CT appearances are consistent with a Stanford type B aortic dissection.

In view of the dissection type, i.e. Stanford type B, the decision is made to manage him conservatively. At outpatient follow-up 3 months later, he is well and normotensive. A follow-up CT scan confirms that the false lumen has occluded.

Case 2

A 70-year-old lady was admitted to the medical ward with an exacerbation of her chronic obstructive pulmonary disease (COPD). Her case was discussed at the weekly unit radiology meeting. Her initial presentation was with pyrexia, a productive cough and slightly increased dyspnoea. The pyrexia and cough had settled with antibiotic therapy but her dyspnoea had continued to worsen, despite bronchodilators, physiotherapy and a trial of steroids.

Initial chest radiograph (on admission)

The heart size and pulmonary vascularity are normal. The lungs are overinflated. Eight anterior ribs are visible in the mid-clavicular line and the hemidiaphragms appear flattened in keeping with the diagnosis of COPD. There was loss of the right hemidiaphragmatic silhouette and an associated area of increased density at the right base. Appearances are consistent with right lower lobe consolidation.

Chest radiograph 3 days later

The appearances are unchanged.

Chest radiograph 2 days later

The right diaphragmatic silhouette remains obscured by the right basal density. In addition there is a meniscus noted peripherally, extending up along the lateral chest wall to the apex. This latter appearance is consistent with a pleural effusion.

The medical registrar then informs the meeting that the clinical appearances were also consistent with a right-sided pleural effusion. He consults the radiologist for advice regarding further imaging and intervention.

Ultrasound chest

A large anechoic (dark) area is noted above the diaphragm with a central echogenic triangular zone. There were no septations visible. The ultrasonic image is consistent with a large pleural effusion. The central zone represents consolidated lung.

Because of the clinical concern regarding underlying malignancy, in consultation with the radiologists, the decision was made to undergo CT of the chest, with a view to possible CT guided drainage.

CT chest

The initial set of images confirm the right lower lobe consolidation, with an associated low attenuation zone peripherally, consistent with the known pleural effusion. No mass lesion or endobronchial stenosis is seen.

The second set demonstrates the patient has been turned into the prone position.

A needle is identified, the tip of which lies in the pleural collection. Subsequent images shown that a wire and finally a 12F pigtail catheter are located within the collection.

The medical registrar informs you that the procedure was routine, and that straw-coloured aspirate was drained. Biochemical and microbiological analysis revealed a sterile exudative pleural effusion. The patient's dyspnoea improved dramatically overnight, and the fluid was sent for cytological evaluation.*

*Cytological evaluation showed no evidence of malignancy. The effusion was para-pneumonic in nature. The patient made an excellent recovery and was discharged.

Case 3

A 24-year-old male patient was transferred from the orthopaedic unit to the medical admissions unit 2 days ago following an episode of haemoptysis.

He had been admitted to hospital 10 days earlier following a fractured right femur sustained when his bicycle had been involved in a road traffic accident with a car. His right femur had been treated by open reduction and internal fixation with an intramedullary nail.

On examination he was dyspnoeic with a tachycardia of 120 bpm. His blood pressure is 103/50. ECG reveals right bundle branch block and a sinus tachycardia. An arterial blood gas sample confirms a type 1 respiratory failure picture with a PaO_2 of 7.9 kPa on 50% oxygen. There is no evidence of an axillary rash.

Chest x-ray

Heart size and pulmonary vascularity are normal. No active lung lesion. Normal chest radiograph.

VQ scan

There is an area of mismatch at the right lung base. Appearances are suspicious of a pulmonary embolus (intermediate/high probability). CT recommended to confirm the diagnosis of pulmonary embolus.

CT scan

A dynamically enhanced multidetector CT scan was performed using the pulmonary angiographic algorithm. The pulmonary conus and main pulmonary arteries enhance normally. A central filling defect is noted in the right descending pulmonary artery. The appearance of this defect—the 'polo-mint' sign—is consistent with a pulmonary embolus in the right descending pulmonary artery.

He is commenced on therapeutic low molecular weight heparin (LMWH) and warfarinized. When the INR was greater than 2.0, his LMWH was discontinued and he was discharged on warfarin with suitable follow-up arrangements in place.

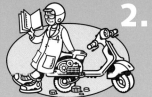

2. Breast Mass or Breast Screening

Focal breast lesions may present in three ways: the mass may be discovered by the patient on self-examination, by a doctor during a clinical examination or as part of a breast-screening programme. Breast screening begins initially with mammography, but may proceed to triple assessment with mammography and ultrasound forming the usual imaging modalities (Fig. 2.1). Furthermore, imaging may be used to guide biopsy either by ultrasound or stereotaxis.

The breast lump

Management of the symptomatic breast lump depends on the patient's age.

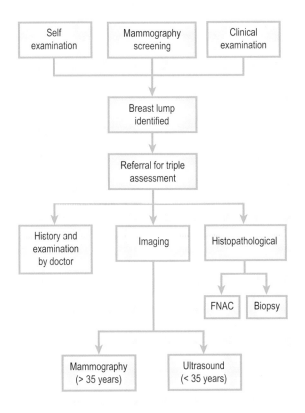

Fig. 2.1 Algorithm for breast lump assessment. (FNA(C), fine needle aspiration (cytology).)

The patient is under 35 years of age

Following clinical examination, the first imaging modality used is ultrasound. If the lesion is cystic, then typically no further intervention is necessary. If the lesion is solid, fine needle aspiration (FNA) is performed. The most common solid mass in this age group is a benign fibroadenoma (see Fig. 20.16).

The patient is 35 years of age or older

The preliminary imaging technique is mammography (using craniocaudal and lateral oblique projections). If a focal mass is identified on the mammogram, then ultrasound of the lesion follows. If the lesion proves cystic, then aspiration is performed. If the lesion is solid on ultrasound (see Fig. 20.17), then FNA is performed. Should mammography identify microcalcification (see Fig. 20.21), then a stereotactic core biopsy of the area is performed to exclude breast carcinoma.

Breast screening

The UK NHS Breast Screening Programme invites women aged from 50 to 69 years of age to attend for breast screening every 3 years.

At screening, two-view (lateral oblique and craniocaudal) mammographic studies of each breast are performed. These radiographs are independently reported by two radiologists. If normal, the patient will be reviewed again in 3 years. This will be the case in 95% of those presenting.

If there is an abnormality on the two-view screening study (see Fig. 20.22), the patient will be recalled to an assessment clinic. Approximately 5% of patients will be recalled to this clinic, where a radiologist, clinician, pathologist, radiographer and breast care nurse will be in attendance. Further radiographic views (coned or magnification views) and/or breast ultrasound will be arranged.

If there is persistent abnormality, e.g. evidence of a solid mass (see Fig. 20.19), parenchymal distortion (see Fig. 20.18) or abnormal patterns of calcification, then image-guided fine needle aspiration (FNA) or core biopsy can be performed. The image guidance used may be ultrasound or stereotactic radiography.

Depending on the pathological outcome, there are three possibilities: surgery, early recall or 3-yearly follow-up. The emphasis in breast screening is to reach a definite diagnosis at the initial assessment clinic so approximately 20% will go to surgery, 80% to 3-year follow-up, and only a very tiny minority (approximately 0.25%) referred for early recall in 6–9 months.

 Breast carcinoma is the second commonest malignancy in women in the UK.

Case conference

 A 54-year-old lady was referred by her general practitioner to the 'one stop breast clinic' with a mass in the upper outer quadrant of her left breast. Her menopause was at the age of 51 years. She has noticed the lump over the past 4 weeks while showering. On examination, a firm, 2 cm, fixed mass was noted in the upper outer quadrant. The contralateral breast and the axillae were unremarkable. Examination of the cervical lymph nodes, abdomen and spine was normal.

Mammogram
Craniocaudal and mediolateral images of the left breast were reviewed. In the upper outer quadrant of the left breast, there is a spiculated lesion with microcalcification.

No other lesion is seen. The appearances are very suspicious of a carcinoma, and ultrasound guided FNA is recommended.

Ultrasound
Under ultrasound guidance, the lesion in the left breast was identified, confirmed to be solid, and biopsied. The cytologist confirmed the radiologist's diagnosis of carcinoma.

Conclusion
Her case was discussed at the weekly multidisciplinary meeting and surgery was scheduled for the following week. A wide location excision and axillary node clearance were undertaken. Adjuvant chemotherapy in the form of anastrozole was commenced.

3. Dysphagia

In dysphagia, clinical examination is of limited value, and generally medical imaging or endoscopy is required to make a definitive diagnosis.

Plain chest radiographs are occasionally able to identify pathology, such as achalasia or a hiatus hernia. The mainstay of imaging is with upper gastrointestinal contrast studies, usually with barium, although on occasion with a water-soluble agent if perforation is suspected (barium causes a severe mediastinitis if it leaks). CT is generally reserved for tumour staging or surveillance. In the case of oesophageal carcinoma, endoluminal ultrasound is a developing area in the assessment of tumour depth, and thus potential for surgery.

PET has a growing role in the staging of oesophageal malignancy.

 A retrosternal thyroid mass is a differential diagnosis for an anterior mediastinal mass on CXR.

 Achalasia is a predisposing factor for oesophageal carcinoma.

There are two main causes of dysphagia: thyroid masses and oesophageal diseases.

Thyroid mass

The chest x-ray (CXR) may show contralateral displacement of the trachea by a thyroid mass (benign or malignant). X-rays of the thoracic inlet (AP and lateral views) will show tracheal displacement and narrowing.

Ultrasound demonstrates enlargement of the thyroid, the size and consistency of focal thyroid masses, and any associated lymphadenopathy.

Isotope thyroid studies will identify 'hot' and 'cold' lesions. 'Cold' lesions have an association with malignancy: for a single nodule, 15–25%; for multiple nodules 1–6%. CT assesses retrosternal extension and, if carcinoma is suspected, lymphadenopathy and metastatic tumour spread.

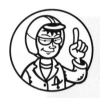 Metastatic pulmonary lesions from thyroid carcinoma produce a 'miliary' appearance on chest x-ray (as may histoplasmosis and TB).

Oesophageal diseases

Oesophageal web
Barium swallow demonstrates a fine anterior transverse filling defect in the upper oesophageal lumen (see Fig. 21.4). Clinical associations of webs include Plummer–Vinson (Paterson–Brown Kelly) syndrome.

Pharyngeal pouch
Barium swallow shows a pouch containing barium and food debris at the upper end of the oesophagus (see Fig. 21.8). The pouch is found at Killian's dehiscence, which is between the thyropharyngeus and cricopharyngeus fibres of the inferior constrictor muscle (see also Ch. 10).

Oesophageal candidiasis
Barium swallow reveals an irregular mucosa with multiple filling defects (see Fig. 21.3). This is more commonly diagnosed at endoscopy.

Achalasia
CXR demonstrates a dilated oesophagus, often with a fluid level. The gastric air bubble is classically absent. There may also be evidence of repeated pulmonary aspiration with fibrotic changes in the dependent lung.

Barium reveals a dilated oesophagus with a smoothly tapering lower end. Irregular stricturing suggests malignant transformation (see Figs 21.1, 21.2).

Hiatus hernia

Chest x-ray demonstrates a retrocardiac air-filled structure, on occasion with a fluid level (see Fig. 21.12). A left lateral film will confirm its location and the diagnosis.

Barium swallow will show the location and the extent of the hernia, and confirm the presence of gastro-oesophageal reflux disease (GORD).

 Hiatus hernias can be subdivided into sliding (80%) and rolling or paraoesophageal hernias (20%).

Oesophageal varices

Although endoscopy is now the primary imaging modality, barium studies reveal serpiginous filling defects along the long axis of the oesophagus, particularly in the prone position (see Fig. 21.6). Ultrasound will show the hepatic architecture, particularly cirrhosis, focal liver lesions, splenomegaly and ascites. CT will confirm the ultrasound findings, as well as aberrant vessels (e.g. splanchnic varices, portal venous transformation, the periumbilical 'caput medusae') and focal liver lesions (e.g. hepatoma).

 Look for associated clinical signs of chronic liver disease, chiefly splenomegaly.

Oesophageal corrosive stricture

This follows ingestion of corrosive liquids. Barium studies show a long smooth tapering stricture (see Fig. 21.5).

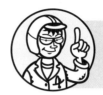 A long, gently tapered stricture is nearly always benign.

Oesophageal carcinoma

CXR is insensitive at diagnosing an oesophageal carcinoma unless the proximal oesophagus is distended, in which case a fluid level may be appreciable. However, pulmonary and skeletal metastases may be appreciated, as may evidence of previous surgery, e.g. total oesophagectomy, in which case there is a widened mediastinum due to the transposed stomach and an absent gastric air bubble in the left hypochondrium.

Barium swallow shows an irregular shouldered stricture—'the rat's tail' (see Fig. 21.7). An associated hiatus hernia suggests that the carcinoma may have resulted from area of Barrett's oesophagus secondary to reflux. This would be an adenocarcinoma. CT is used to stage the disease and identify nodes, tumour fixity and metastatic spread. PET scanning is gaining increased acceptance as the staging test for oesophageal disease. Endoluminal ultrasound is helpful in assessing the depth of tumour invasion.

 A history of chronic reflux with Barrett's oesophagus is significant in the development of adenocarcinoma of the lower third of the oesophagus.

Case conference

A 68-year-old lady presented to the gastroenterologists with a 3-month history of increasingly progressive dysphagia. She had lost 10 kg in weight. She has an extensive smoking history. On examination, she was cachexic. No fasciculations were seen and cranial nerves were intact.

CXR
Cardiac contour and pulmonary vascularity are normal. There is an area of scarring at the right apex. No other pulmonary abnormality is seen.

Barium swallow
There is a 4 cm long strictured area with loss of the normal oesophageal mucosa. 'Shouldering' is noted at the edges of the stricture. Barium passes beyond the stricture into the distal oesophagus and stomach. The stomach and duodenum outline normally. The appearances are consistent with an oesophageal carcinoma.

CT scan
A dynamically enhanced multidetector CT scan was performed through the chest and upper abdomen. There is dilatation of the upper oesophagus with an abrupt change in calibre at the level of the carina, corresponding to an endoscopic level of 28 cm. Fat planes are preserved around the oesophagus. There are two nodes present in the mediastinum, both less than 1 cm in diameter. An area of fibrotic parenchymal scarring is identified in the right upper lobe bronchus. There was no definite pulmonary mass lesion.

Within the abdomen the liver, adrenal glands, pancreas, spleen and kidneys are normal. There is no significant adenopathy or ascites.

Conclusion
The appearances are consistent with an oesophageal mass lesion. Two mediastinal lymph nodes are identified, as is an area of fibrosis in the right upper lobe. The abdomen is normal. PET–CT is recommended for further staging.

PET–CT scan
A whole body PET–CT scan was performed following the IV administration of ^{18}FDG. A glucose-avid lesion is identified in the oesophagus at the level of the carina. There is no isotope uptake in the mediastinum or right apex. No other glucose-avid lesion is demonstrated.

The appearances are consistent with an oesophageal carcinoma. There is no evidence of disease outside the oesophagus.

She is referred back to the gastroenterologists for consideration for surgery.

4. Abdominal Pain

Imaging in abdominal pain

The differential diagnosis for abdominal pain is immense. There are many imaging tests at one's disposal. The judicious use of these will depend on a thorough patient examination, and the clinical impression of the underlying pathology will dictate the imaging direction, e.g. loin pain and haematuria—urological; right upper quadrant pain in an overweight 43-year-old lady—hepatobiliary; central abdominal pain radiating to the back in an arteriopath—aortic aneurysm.

Plain abdominal radiographs are useful for evaluating gas, both intraluminal and extraluminal, and calculi.

Ultrasound is sensitive in the evaluation of any fluid-filled structure, excellent at detecting calculi and good at evaluation of solid organs. A kidney obstructed by calculus with a resultant hydronephrosis is elegantly demonstrated by ultrasound. On the other hand, ultrasound is very insensitive in the evaluation of gaseous structures, as the sound waves are reflected by air. Searching for a duodenal ulcer with ultrasound is a fruitless task!

Computed tomography (CT) has all the advantages of plain radiographs and ultrasound. So, why not use it for everything? The radiation dose generated by CT is large and must be clinically justified.

The likelihood of anyone contracting a malignancy from the Earth's background radiation is 1:1,000,000. Following a CT of the abdomen, this rises to 1:2000. Furthermore, the risk rises with successive scans, no matter whether they are performed the next day or 20 years later. On the other hand, the risk of contracting a malignancy during one's life is 1:3. It all comes down to relative risk. How sick is the patient? How old is the patient? Can the imaging be acquired by alternative methodology, e.g. ultrasound, MRI or endoscopy?

Systems which cause abdominal pain are:
- Intestinal.
- Hepatopancreatobiliary.
- Urological.
- Vascular.
- Gynaecological.
- Miscellaneous.

Intestinal causes

- Large bowel obstruction.
- Small bowel obstruction.
- Volvulus.
- Pseudo-obstruction.
- Diverticulosis.
- Pneumoperitoneum.
- Intestinal ischaemia.
- Appendicitis.

Large bowel obstruction

On the abdominal x-ray (AXR) there are dilated large bowel loops, with haustral markings evident, which occupy a peripheral location on the film (see Fig. 21.22). A cut-off point may be apparent, as may small bowel dilatation, if there is an associated incompetent ileocaecal valve.

Contrast studies will identify the level of bowel obstruction. Barium is used primarily unless there is a significant risk of perforation in which case water-soluble contrast, such as gastrograffin or iopamidol (Niopam), may be substituted. CT will demonstrate change in bowel calibre and the level of obstruction. The underlying aetiology such as a colonic mass may be identified (Fig. 4.1). In such cases, lymphadenopathy and metastatic disease can also be excluded.

Polyp size and malignant transformation	
Size (cm)	Risk of malignant transformation
<0.5	Rarely malignant
<1	1%
1–2	10%
>2	50%

Fig. 4.1 Polyp size and malignant transformation.

Small bowel obstruction

The AXR demonstrates dilated small bowel loops and these occupy a central position on the film (see Fig. 21.15). Valvulae conniventes will be evident, confirming the small bowel nature of the loops. The number of loops is dependent on the level of obstruction within small bowel (e.g. few loops in a high, proximal obstruction). Fluid levels are present on the erect AXR (see Fig. 21.16). A small bowel series with dilute barium identifies the level of obstruction, although if complete obstruction is suspected, a water-soluble contrast such as iopamidol may be more appropriate. CT identifies the level of the obstruction and may determine the likely aetiology, e.g. Crohn's disease with a stricture and inflammatory changes in the surrounding fatty tissues.

The commonest causes of small bowel obstruction are adhesions, hernias and lesions *outside* the small bowel—look for abdominal surgery scars and check the hernial orifices. The commonest causes of large bowel obstruction are adhesions, lesions *inside* the large bowel and hernias.

Volvulus

Volvulus occurs when a loop of gastrointestinal tract twists about its mesentery. The commonest sites are at the stomach, the caecum and the sigmoid colon. Gastric volvulus is described according to the axis of the 'twist' and is classified as organoaxial or mesenteroaxial. Presentation is with epigastric or chest pain.

Caecal volvulus obstructs the terminal ileum, so presents as a small bowel obstruction (Fig. 21.15).

The caecum often lies in the left or right hypochondrium and is absent from its normal location ('empty caecum' sign). Sigmoid volvulus, which characteristically occurs in the more elderly population, presents as a large bowel obstruction (see Fig. 21.23). The twisted loops of the sigmoid colon converge about its mesentery ('coffee-bean' sign). Contrast enema will confirm the sigmoid obstruction, and has a characteristic appearance—the 'bird of prey' sign.

Pseudo-obstruction

AXR identifies small and large bowel dilatation, with no cut-off point. This often follows surgery. A contrast study of the colon will confirm the lack of a 'cut-off' point.

Diverticulosis

The AXR is usually normal. There may be evidence of the complications of diverticular disease, e.g. large bowel obstruction or perforation. The radiological investigation of choice is a contrast enema. Contrast collects in bowel outpouchings (diverticula) (see Fig. 21.17). Evidence of complications, such as stricture and perforation, are also detectable. CT not only confirms the enema findings, but also allows the anatomical delineation of complications (fistulae, strictures, abscess) and image-guided drainage of collections.

Diverticula protrude *outside* the bowel wall and can fill with contrast. Polyps protrude *inside* the bowel lumen and cause a filling defect within the contrast.

Comparison of radiological features of small and large bowel obstruction		
Radiological feature	Small bowel obstruction	Large bowel obstruction
Bowel diameter	<5 cm	>5 cm
Location	Central	Peripheral
Haustra	No	Yes
Valvulae	Yes	No
Large bowel gas	No	Yes, look for 'cut-off'

Fig. 4.2 Comparison of radiological features of small and large bowel obstruction.

Pneumoperitoneum

On the erect chest or abdominal radiograph, free gas is seen beneath the hemidiaphragm(s). On a supine abdominal projection, various radiological signs have been described. These include the falciform ligament sign and Rigler's sign (see Figs 21.9–21.11).

A water-soluble contrast study may detect the leakage of contrast through the perforated bowel wall; however, with a duodenal ulcer, the perforation may quickly be sealed by omentum. A negative study therefore does not exclude the diagnosis. Endoscopy is the investigation of choice. USS will identify free fluid, especially in the subhepatic and pelvic areas. A CT scan will confirm an extravisceral collection, especially useful if the perforation has sealed.

The commonest viscera to perforate are the duodenum (ulcer) and the sigmoid colon (diverticulum).

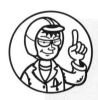

Be aware of Chilaiditi's sign— gas beneath the diaphragm which on close inspection has haustral markings and represents normal intraluminal bowel air, not a perforation.

Causes of pneumoperitoneum: perforated viscus, post laparotomy/oscopy.

Intestinal ischaemia

The AXR demonstrates bowel distension and 'thumbprinting' (see Fig. 21.24). However, 'thumbprinting' is not a specific sign of bowel ischaemia. The splenic flexure is the commonest site in ischaemic colitis. With disease progression, mural and portal venous gas may be appreciated on plain radiographs, the latter sign being very ominous. CT will confirm these features. Other associated pathology may be identified, such as vascular calcification, thrombosis, ascites and visceral perforation.

Appendicitis

On the AXR an appendicolith is seen as a radio-opacity in the right lower quadrant. This finding is present in 14% of cases. US can be used to measure the appendiceal diameter (normal<6 mm) and occasionally to view an appendicolith. This is of particular value in children and young adults. Although CT is not often clinically indicated in these patients, an appendicolith is seen as an intraluminal appendicular calcified mass. Appendicular thickening, inflammation of the surrounding fat planes and free intraperitoneal fluid can also be appreciated.

Appendicitis is essentially a clinical diagnosis.

Contrast studies are contraindicated in intestinal ischaemia due to the risk of bowel perforation.

Hepatopancreatobiliary diseases

- Cholelithiasis.
- Acute pancreatitis.
- Chronic pancreatitis.
- Biliary colic.

Cholelithiasis and biliary colic

Calcified gallstones are seen in the right upper quadrant on AXR in 10–20% of cases as laminated structures of varying size (see Fig. 22.10). US is the investigation of choice, with gallstones seen as bright (echogenic) structures with an associated dark posterior band (the acoustic shadow, Fig. 4.3). Any biliary dilatation will also be evident. The diameter of the common hepatic duct at the porta hepatis is typically ≤6 mm. However it is known to enlarge by 1 mm per decade after 40 years of age, and also is larger in patients with a previous history of cholecystectomy.

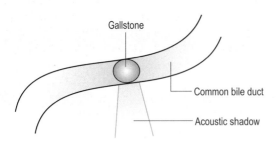

Fig. 4.3 Ultrasound of a stone in the bile duct, showing the acoustic shadow effect.

CT may demonstrate the calculus (if its attenuation value is higher than bile) and any significant biliary dilatation. Other complications of obstructing biliary calculus, e.g. pancreatitis with glandular enlargement, surrounding inflammatory changes and ascites, will be identified.

On MRI, gallstones appear as low signal within the high signal gallbladder bile on T2 weighted (T2W) sequences. Magnetic resonance cholangiography (MRC) superbly visualizes duct calibre and has the advantage of no associated radiation (see Fig. 22.21). ERCP should now be reserved for interventional cases, such as sphincterotomy, stone removal and stent placement (see Fig. 22.9).

Acute pancreatitis

On AXR a sentinel loop and 'cut-off' sign are classically seen. The underlying cause may be apparent, e.g. gallstones.

Ultrasound will detect gallstones, as well as any increase in size or irregularity of the pancreas, although the pancreas can be difficult to view due to obscuring bowel gas. Complications of pancreatitis, including pseudocyst and ascites, are detectable. CT will demonstrate an enlarged and/or oedematous pancreas. Necrosis and pancreatic pseudocysts are clearly outlined (see Figs 22.4, 22.5).

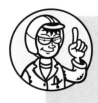

The US identification of gallstones is frequently coincidental. It may not explain the patient's symptomatology. Clinical correlation is paramount.

CT needs to be performed with IV contrast enhancement to detect pancreatic necrosis.

Chronic pancreatitis

The AXR demonstrates speckled calcification transversely across the upper abdomen in the pancreatic distribution (see Fig. 22.6). CT shows pancreatic calcification, along with atrophy of the gland and a dilated pancreatic duct. MRC demonstrates pancreatic duct morphology.

Urological diseases

- Renal colic.
- Renal malignancy.
- Urinary tract infection.

Renal colic

The incidence of renal calculus is 7 per 1000 of the population, with an overall lifetime risk of 40–60% (male : female ratio 2 : 1). Renal calculi are visible on plain abdominal radiographs in up to 60% of cases. Other evidence of the underlying cause, e.g. hyperparathyroidism, may be present, i.e. osteopenic vertebral bodies and vascular calcification. The intravenous urogram (IVU) has traditionally been the gold standard in identifying the presence of calculus and level of ureteric obstruction. The obstructed kidney opacifies later than the normal side. There is delayed filling of the pelvicalyceal system and the calyces are swollen and blunted ('clubbed').

Ultrasound scan, as with gallstones, shows the calculus with its posterior acoustic shadowing but is sensitive in only 40–60% of cases. Calyceal dilatation may be seen proximal to the obstructing calculus. Unenhanced CT identifies renal calculus in 99% of cases. Dilatation of the renal tract proximal to the calculus may be evident. CT urography is gaining acceptance as the first-line investigation in renal colic.

Beware of phleboliths on abdominal radiographs. These are small, smooth, circular venous calcifications. Classically they lie below the level of the ischial spines.

Never comment on an IVU without the preliminary ('control') film.

Renal malignancy

The commonest renal malignancy is renal cell carcinoma. Rarely the AXR may show displacement of adjacent structures, e.g. bowel, by the tumour. Evidence of metastatic bony involvement may be seen as lucent, expansile deposits within the bones. However, the AXR appearances are often normal.

US typically reveals a solid renal mass. Tumour extension into the renal vein and inferior vena cava may be delineated, as may liver metastases. CT demonstrates a solid renal mass (see Fig. 22.7b) and any extension into adjacent structures, particularly the renal vein and inferior vena cava. CT is the gold standard for tumour staging.

If renal malignancy is detected, obtain a chest radiograph to exclude cannonball metastases.

If left-sided testicular varicocoele is the primary diagnosis, check for renal malignancy on USS. The left gonadal vein drains into the left renal vein and can be obstructed by invading left-sided renal tumour.

Urinary tract infection

This is essentially a clinical diagnosis. US is used to look for any underlying cause—calculus, obstruction, evidence of chronicity, scarring or cortical thinning. Nuclear medicine (DMSA) scans are useful for differential renal function and demonstrating renal scarring (see also Ch. 12), and DTPA renograms for excluding renal outlet obstruction.

Vascular diseases

- Abdominal aortic aneurysm.
- Aortic dissection.
- Intestinal ischaemia.

Abdominal aortic aneurysm

The AXR may demonstrate an aneurysm as a curvilinear central or paravertebral calcification with loss of parallelism of the aortic walls (Fig. 4.4). Look for calcification of other vessels. USS

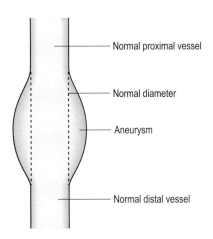

Normal proximal vessel

Normal diameter

Aneurysm

Normal distal vessel

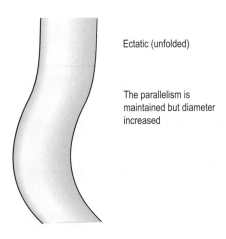

Ectatic (unfolded)

The parallelism is maintained but diameter increased

Fig. 4.4 The difference between an ectatic and an aneurysmal aorta.

23

can accurately measure the transverse dimensions of the aneurysm and the relationship to the neck of the renal arteries (supra-, juxta- and infrarenal). Evidence of para-aortic rupture is detectable.

Contrast enhanced CT is the gold standard for measuring aneurysm dimensions, assessing the relationship with the renal arteries, the nature of the aneurysm (fusiform, saccular) and the calibre of the iliac vessels distal to the aneurysm (Fig. 4.5). It is the gold standard for identifying an aortic leak. Helical and multidetector (multislice) CT imaging is important in the planning of aortic stent patients (Fig. 4.6; see also Fig. 20.11).

Aortic dissection

CT delineates the origin and length of the dissection and identifies the true and false aneurysm lumina. It confirms renal and visceral artery patency and perfusion. Dissections are typically thoracic in origin so it is necessary to scan from the origin of the great arch vessels to the femoral arteries (Fig. 4.7; see also Ch. 1). Many centres perform an unenhanced scan first to look for mural haematoma and to distinguish slow flow in a false lumen from mural thrombus.

Intestinal ischaemia

See above, page 21.

Gynaecological diseases

Ectopic pregnancy

US shows free fluid within the pouch of Douglas and an empty uterus.

An adnexal mass may also be evident (see Ch. 15).

Fibroids (leiomyomata)

The AXR may show a discrete calcified pelvic lesion. US identifies discrete, solid, hypoechoic and sometimes multiple uterine masses. On MRI, simple fibroids are seen as discrete, solid, low signal masses on T1W and T2W sequences. Heterogeneous areas of high signal on the T2W are associated with fibroid degeneration.

Torsion of ovarian cyst

US will demonstrate pelvic free fluid and an adnexal cystic mass.

Endometriosis

US is used first line to detect the solid and cystic mass(es) of endometriosis. These are seen most commonly on the ovary and broad ligament. Chocolate cysts (endometriomas) on MRI have a distinct signal pattern due to the blood breakdown products.

Normal aortic diameter	
Vertebral level	Normal aortic diameter (cm)
T12	2.5
L2	2.0
L4	1.5

Fig. 4.5 Normal aortic diameter.

Stanford classification of thoracic aortic dissection		
Type	Origin	Treatment
A	Ascending aortic arch	Surgical
B	Distal to subclavian artery	Conservative

Fig. 4.7 Stanford classification of thoracic aortic dissection.

Surveillance of AAA	
Maximum aneurysm diameter (cm)	Action
3.5–4.5	Annual US scan
4.6–5.5	6-monthly US scan review
>5.5	Consider surgery/endovascular repair

Fig. 4.6 Surveillance of AAA.

Abdominal/pelvic abscess

Displacement of adjacent structures can be seen on AXR and air fluid levels on erect films. US demonstrates cystic and complex fluid collections and is useful for planning guided intervention. CT outlines the same features as US but may also indicate associated pathology or cause, e.g. diverticular disease, pancreatitis.

Pelvic inflammatory disease

This is primarily a clinical diagnosis in women of childbearing age. US is used to exclude complications, e.g. hydrosalpinx and pyosalpinx.

Transvaginal US gives better image resolution of the uterus and ovaries than transabdominal US, but is a more invasive (and intimate) examination.

Case conferences

Case 1
A 56-year-old woman presented on last night's take with abdominal pain and vomiting that she had had for about a week, gradually getting worse. She has a history of surgery for removal of a carcinoid tumour of the terminal ileum 5 years previously. She has been well ever since.

Plain radiographs
Abdominal radiographs demonstrate multiple distended loops of bowel. These are located centrally within the abdomen, and the presence of valvulae conniventes confirms them as small bowel loops. There is no gas in the colon or rectum.

The appearances are consistent with mechanical small bowel obstruction.

Small bowel series
There are distended loops of small bowel. There was no progression of contrast into the large bowel. The appearances are consistent with mechanical small bowel obstruction.

CT abdomen
CT of the abdomen with IV contrast demonstrates an irregular mass lesion in the right iliac fossa invading the adjacent bowel mesentery. Distended loops of small bowel are confirmed. Large bowel diameter is normal. There are multiple low attenuation lesions within both lobes of the liver.

The appearances are consistent with a malignant tumour mass invading the mesentery and causing small bowel obstruction. There are also multiple liver metastases.

Given the known history of terminal ileal carcinoid, the diagnosis could be confirmed by octreotide (sandostatin) nuclear medicine imaging.

Case 2

A 53-year-old lady was referred by her general practitioner with a 7-month history of lower abdominal pain and intermittent vaginal bleeding. She had been climacteric for the past 14 months. History was otherwise unremarkable. No significant abnormality was found on abdominal examination. Per vaginal examination: no mass lesion or discharge noted.

Abdominal radiograph

The bowel gas pattern is unremarkable with no evidence of intestinal obstruction or perforation. There is no evidence of renal or ureteric calculi. A 4 cm circular calcific density is noted centrally within the pelvis.

Ultrasound of abdomen and pelvis

The gallbladder, liver, biliary tree and pancreas outline normally. Both kidneys are sonographically normal with no evidence of calculus, hydronephrosis or mass lesion.

Above the bladder, the uterus is prominent and there is a 4 cm mass with posterior acoustic shadowing noted within it. The appearances are consistent with those seen on the abdominal radiograph, and are very suggestive of a calcified fibroid.

MR pelvis

Axial, sagittal and coronal T2W sequences, along with sagittal T1W and STIR (fat suppression), are available for review. There is a focal mass measuring 4.1 cm in diameter seen within the dorsal uterine wall on all sequences. The characteristics are of a low signal lesion on all pulse sequences, and the appearance is consistent with a uterine fibroid. No other significant abnormality is seen.

This lady's gynaecologist informed her of these reassuring findings and management options. She chose medical management with follow-up at outpatients.

5. Jaundice

Jaundice is a presenting symptom crossing medical and surgical specialties, its underlying causes ranging from the entirely reversible (biliary calculi) to the fatal (pancreatic cancer). It is in delineating these pathologies that imaging has a pivotal role—establishing the aetiology and thus the correct treatment modality. Increasingly the radiologist has the primary interventional role in the management of hepatobiliary malignancies.

There are several imaging investigations available for the assessment of the jaundiced patient and a logical sequence in which to use them based on clinical and biochemical findings. Ultrasound, CT, MRC and PTC are all helpful in different ways, supplemented by ERCP which has both a diagnostic and a therapeutic role. The choice of initial investigation should be guided by clinical acumen. The middle aged, overweight, Caucasian lady with right upper quadrant pain is likely to have gallstone disease, making ultrasound appropriate initially. On the other hand, a 75-year-old man with deep, painless jaundice, 10 kg of weight loss and an elevated CA 19-9 tumour marker is more likely to require a CT abdomen to exclude pancreatic carcinoma.

Liver diseases

Hepatitis
On ultrasound, acute hepatitis generally has no distinguishing features. Chronic hepatitis has appearances similar to cirrhosis.

Cirrhosis
Radiologically, the appearances reflect two stages in the disease: fatty change and fibrosis. A fatty liver is enlarged or normal in size. On ultrasound, fatty liver is coarse with decreased penetration and, when fibrotic, is shrunken with an irregular margin. CT of the fatty liver shows an enlarged, low attenuation (dark) organ. In advanced disease, the liver becomes small. The margins may be irregular, and sparing of the caudate lobe is characteristic. In chronic cirrhosis, careful evaluation of the liver must be made for a focal hepatic mass, i.e. a regenerating nodule or, more worryingly, the development of a hepatocellular carcinoma.

The focal liver lesion
There are six commonly occurring liver lesions which, although not necessarily associated with jaundice, constitute a significant proportion of a radiologist's working practice. A detailed description of these is beyond the scope of this book, but some basic principles apply.

The lesions are (see Fig. 22.15):
- Simple hepatic cyst.
- Haemangioma.
- Hepatic adenoma.
- Focal nodular hyperplasia.
- Hepatocellular carcinoma.
- Metastases.

Simple hepatic cyst
This is the most common focal hepatic 'mass' detected. On ultrasound, it is completely dark ('anechoic'), with a bright tail ('through enhancement') deep to it. It is of low attenuation on CT (<15 Hounsfield units) and does not enhance with IV contrast. On MR a cyst is of low signal on T1W and high signal on T2W sequences. Its signal will be identical to the CSF within the spinal canal.

Haemangioma
A common incidental finding in cross-sectional imaging studies and on ultrasound, a haemangioma is typically brighter (hyperechoic) than the surrounding liver parenchyma. On unenhanced CT, haemangiomas are of lower attenuation (i.e. darker) than the surrounding liver. However, within a few minutes of contrast administration, they show a nodular, peripheral enhancement which, within 15–30 minutes, will be uniform and obscure the mass from the surrounding liver. T1W post-contrast MR sequences demonstrate the same 'centripetal' enhancement, but the lesion remains brighter than the surrounding liver. A further characteristic MR feature of a haemangioma is that the lesions remain

very bright on long T2W sequences. This has been termed the 'lightbulb' sign.

Hepatic adenoma

This mass occurs in younger women and has an association with the oral contraceptive pill. It is usually symptomatic (the patient has abdominal pain) and is the result of bleeding from within the adenoma. This bleeding and the presence of fat within the lesion have particular MR signal characteristics that allow the diagnosis to be made.

Focal nodular hyperplasia (FNH)

Often an asymptomatic incidental finding, FNH represents normal hepatocytes and Kupffer cells, arranged abnormally. An arteriovenous malformation may form the central nidus. Approximately 50% have a central scar. It is typically hypoechoic on ultrasound. MR characteristics are similar to the surrounding liver (unlike hepatic adenoma) on T1W and T2W sequences. The lesion typically enhances promptly on MR, but the scar characteristically shows delayed enhancement.

Hepatocellular carcinoma (HCC)

Hepatocellular carcinoma often occurs in association with underlying liver problems, e.g. viral hepatitis, cirrhosis or alcoholic liver disease. For this reason those with established cirrhosis should be enrolled in a hepatocellular carcinoma ultrasound surveillance programme. A knowledge of the history and background imaging findings can be very helpful in making the diagnosis. Elevation of serum alpha-fetoprotein is characteristic, except in those with the fibrolamellar variant—younger patients with normal livers.

Hepatocellular carcinoma is solitary in 50% of cases, multifocal in 20% and diffuse in 30%. A surrounding capsule, internal septa, daughter nodules and tumour thrombus in adjacent veins are helpful diagnostic features.

On CT, the tumour is seen as a low attenuation mass within the liver. Arterial phase enhancement is seen, both on CT and MRI. Central areas of necrosis are characteristic. On nuclear medicine studies, uptake of gallium 67 (Ga^{67}) occurs within the mass, whereas with technetium^{99m} (Tc^{99m}) sulphur colloid, isotope is taken up by the surrounding liver, not the tumour.

Metastases

Occasionally, liver metastases can calcify, e.g. colloid colorectal metastases, and therefore can be identified on the abdominal radiograph. Usually, however, the diagnosis of metastatic disease requires cross-sectional imaging. On ultrasound, the appearances are of dark (hypoechoic) circular solid areas within the liver. On CT, these dark areas are of low attenuation. On MR, liver metastases are typically of lower signal on T1W, and of higher signal on T2W sequences, than the surrounding liver. A useful rule on MR is that the signal characteristics of liver metastatic lesions are the same as the spleen.

Hydatid disease

Plain films may show liver calcification, oval or circular being typical; ultrasound (and MR) will confirm the cystic nature of the lesion and the presence of daughter cysts. CT will localize the disease and define the extent.

Biliary diseases

Gallstones
See Chapter 4.

Cholangiocarcinoma

Cholangiocarcinoma is an adenocarcinoma that arises from bile duct epithelium. It is classified as intra- or extrahepatic. Intrahepatic cholangiocarcinomas are further differentiated by location into hilar (Klatskin tumours) or peripheral. Peripheral is defined as being distal to the second bifurcation of the left or right hepatic duct.

Peripheral cholangiocarcinoma
This is usually seen on CT and MR as a large, well-defined, lobular mass, with peripheral enhancement on both modalities.

Hilar cholangiocarcinoma (the Klatskin tumour)
Hilar cholangiocarcinoma represents more than 50% of large bile duct cancers. The most common presentation (>70%) is as a small infiltrating tumour. Because of the location, jaundice is an early presenting feature. CT may demonstrate a thickened, high attenuation duct wall which occludes the lumen.

Extrahepatic cholangiocarcinoma

The cardinal feature on US, CT and MR studies is the demonstration of biliary dilatation proximal to the lesion, and of normal calibre distal to it. The lesion itself can be located at the level of the bile duct's diameter transition. Contrast examinations, e.g. PTC or ERCP, will identify the level of the disease as a biliary stricture. Both techniques permit subsequent therapeutic intervention and cytological evaluation.

Ulcerative colitis is a risk factor for the development of cholangiocarcinoma.

Bile duct strictures

Benign bile duct strictures are the result of trauma, surgery, ERCP, inflammatory processes, infections and cholangitis, either primary sclerosing or Asiatic. US, CT and MR (MRC) will confirm the biliary dilatation. MRC in particular is useful in determining the level of any stricture. Sclerosing cholangitis has a characteristic 'beaded' appearance of the biliary tree on MRC.

Pancreatic carcinoma

On both US and CT, pancreatic adenocarcinoma appears as a darker mass within the gland (see Fig. 22.7). CT delineates the lesion more effectively, can confirm biliary and/or pancreatic ductal dilatation, atrophy of the distal gland, tumour infiltration into the surrounding structures (particularly tumour involvement of the mesenteric and portal vessels), lymphadenopathy and metastatic spread. Both US and CT permit image-guided biopsy.

If multiple hepatic cysts are seen, assess the kidneys for polycystic kidney disease.

Beading of the biliary tree is characteristic of primary sclerosing cholangitis—check for a history of associated ulcerative colitis.

Case conference

An 82-year-old man was referred to the hepatobiliary surgeons with a 3-month history of vague abdominal pain, anorexia and 5 kg weight loss. He had a past medical history of three myocardial infarctions and emphysema. On clinical examination he was noted to be jaundiced, and biochemical evaluation confirmed cholestatic jaundice. His CA 19-9 marker was noted to be significantly elevated.

Abdominal radiograph
The gas pattern is unremarkable. There is no evidence of intestinal obstruction or perforation.

Minor degenerative changes are noted in the lumbar vertebrae, but there is no evidence of metastatic disease.

Ultrasound of abdomen
The gallbladder is distended and no stones are visible. The common hepatic duct is significantly dilated at 1.4 cm. There is intrahepatic duct dilatation. Multiple hypoechoic lesions measuring approximately 1 cm are noted within the liver. The pancreas is obscured by gas. No other abnormality is seen.

CT chest and abdomen
In the chest there are multiple lesions seen within both lungs. The liver also contains multiple low attenuation lesions, and the biliary dilatation is confirmed. There is a 4 cm low attenuation mass in the head of the pancreas. Dilatation of the distal pancreatic duct and atrophy of the distal gland are also noted. The mass abuts the mesenteric vessels, with loss of the fat plane between them. The appearances are consistent with a pancreatic carcinoma with evidence of local invasion. There are liver and lung metastases.

In view of the advanced nature of the disease, and the patient's general health, palliation was performed by placing a biliary stent endoscopically at ERCP. Following this, the patient's jaundice resolved quickly. He was discharged to the care of his family, general practitioner and palliative care team. He demised 6 weeks later.

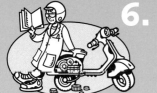

6. Altered Bowel Habit/Rectal Bleeding

Altered bowel habit is a common gastrointestinal presenting complaint. Faeces containing blood, fresh or changed, is by definition, altered.

Imaging should be considered only after a full history and an appropriate assessment, including per rectum (PR) examination. Not all patients will warrant radiological assistance for diagnosis—haemorrhoids and irritable bowel syndrome, for example, are clinical diagnoses (albeit the latter established by exclusion). However, at times imaging can reassure both the patient and clinician. Those that do justify further investigation may benefit from imaging in isolation or, more commonly, in conjunction with endoscopic studies. Consideration should be given to the urgency of the clinical presentation. An acutely unwell hospital admission with suspected small bowel obstruction will require immediate attention, whereas a chronic history of altered bowel habit may be undertaken as an outpatient with follow up at clinic.

Plain AXRs are a sensible starting point for many patients, most importantly to exclude obstruction or perforation, and are frequently requested for non-specific abdominal pain. Following these, contrast studies are the next likely imaging step, although CT is increasingly used, including the technique of CT colonography.

The exclusion of colorectal carcinoma (CRC), diverticular and inflammatory bowel disease (IBD) forms a substantial proportion of those patients attending with altered bowel habit and PR bleeding. Of course, these pathologies can coexist, making interpretation more of a challenge. In the case of CRC, ulcerative colitis (UC) and diverticular disease, a contrast enema is the imaging investigation of choice. For Crohn's disease, a small bowel series is more appropriate, as the terminal ileum is the most frequently affected area. A barium enema should be considered if there is suspicion of large bowel Crohn's disease.

Crohn's disease is asymmetrical and discontinuous; ulcerative colitis is symmetrical and continuous.

In a limited number of cases, more specialist imaging studies are useful. A radiolabelled white cell scan proves helpful in delineating the extent of inflamed or affected bowel in IBD. Those with persistent or significant PR bleeding may benefit from a radiolabelled red cell scan or mesenteric angiography—most valuably in those bleeding acutely—to identify a focal source.

Angiodysplasia and irritable bowel syndrome are both diagnoses of exclusion.

Double contrast enema produces excellent large bowel mucosal detail.

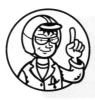

A labelled red cell scan essentially requires active bleeding at the time of investigation.

Small bowel diseases

Crohn's disease
The plain abdominal x-ray may be unremarkable, but can show, on occasion, intestinal obstruction or evidence of toxic megacolon. It is important to review the sacroiliac (SI) joints for evidence of sacroiliitis (see Ch. 9).

The hallmarks of Crohn's disease are that it is most common at the terminal ileum, is asymmetrical and discontinuous. On small bowel

Fig. 6.1 The features of Crohn's disease.

barium studies, i.e. small bowel series or enema (enteroclysis), look for 'rose-thorn' and aphthoid ulcers, thickened blunted valvulae conniventes, cobblestoning, strictures ('string sign of Kantor'; see Fig. 21.14), bowel loop separation and pseudosacculations. Large bowel features are similar (see Fig. 6.1).

Scleroderma

Scleroderma is a systemic disorder. Malabsorption may follow small bowel involvement. On barium studies, the bowel is hypomobile or atonic, and the lumen, diffusely enlarged, has thickened mucosal folds and pseudosacculations. It is said to have a 'hidebound' appearance. Similarly, the large bowel is atonic with pseudosacculations on the antimesenteric border.

Coeliac disease

Barium examination demonstrates jejunal dilatation but normal fold thickness. The number of jejunal folds decreases and the ileal folds increase. This reversal ('flip-flop' pattern) occurs with chronic disease. On the small bowel barium examination there is segmentation of the barium. The 'moulage' sign—a wax cast appearance of barium in a featureless tube—is due to the complete effacement of the mucosal folds. Coeliac disease may be complicated by lymphoma.

Large bowel diseases

Colorectal cancer

Plain abdominal radiographs may be normal in the absence of intestinal obstruction, in which case there is evidence typically of small bowel obstruction with right sided tumours, and of large bowel obstruction with left-sided lesions.

In the well-prepared patient, double contrast barium enema (DCBE) should allow excellent visualization of the colorectal mucosa. All non-mobile filling defects must be viewed with suspicion, as colorectal cancers evolve from polyps (see Fig. 21.18). Radiologically, there are two chief forms of colorectal cancer on DCBE: 'apple-core' strictures (usually left-sided) and ulcerating or linear masses involving one wall of the bowel (usually right-sided; see Fig. 21.20).

Conditions predisposing to colorectal cancer include:
- Familial adenoma polyposis coli.
- Hereditary non-polyposis colorectal cancer.
- Gardner's syndrome (associated with osteomas of skull and mandible and desmoids of mesentery).
- Inflammatory bowel disease.

Approximately half of all colorectal cancers arise within 20 cm of the anal margin. As the sigmoid colon can be very tortuous, this, in the presence of diverticular disease—endemic in the over 60s—necessitates careful evaluation.

Familial polyposis coli is a genetically transmitted (autosomal dominant) colorectal carcinomatous disease which presents in the second or third decade of life. Radiological manifestations on DCBE are of thousands of polyps 'carpeting' the colonic mucosa (see Fig. 21.19). Associated disorders include Gardner's syndrome, in which polyposis is found with osteomas of the mandible. Like polyposis coli, it is autosomal dominant.

CT is the mainstay of staging and will exclude lymphadenopathy, liver metastatic disease, the presence of adjacent visceral involvement, such as that of the bladder and ureter, and the tumour itself. CT colonography is an imaging method gaining increased acceptance in the diagnosis of colorectal polyps. The patient, having taken a standard bowel preparation to cleanse the colon, undergoes standard bowel insufflation with a rectal catheter. CT of the abdomen and pelvis is performed in both the prone and supine positions. Polyps and masses, unlike faecal residue, should be fixed, regardless of patient positioning.

The role of MR is currently being evaluated as an imaging tool in rectal cancer. Unlike CT, the layers of the rectal wall can be delineated, and therefore local disease staging, particularly mesorectal involvement, can be performed and the need for adjuvant therapy evaluated. Some centres currently use endoanal ultrasound to evaluate the depth of tumour involvement in anorectal cancer.

CT colonography is particularly useful in infirm patients who are unable to undergo colonoscopy or barium enema.

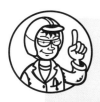

In familial polyposis coli total colectomy with ileorectal anastomosis or ileostomy is usually undertaken before 20 years of age before carcinoma develops.

Colorectal cancers are glucose avid following ¹⁸FDG (fluorodeoxyglucose) administration. PET imaging is therefore very useful in staging the tumour and quantitating tumour recurrence and metastatic disease.

Diverticular disease
See Chapter 4.

Ulcerative colitis
Important AXR findings are toxic megacolon, which is seen in ≤10% of cases (see Fig. 21.25). Sacroiliitis may also be noted. The hallmark of this disease on contrast studies is that it is, unlike Crohn's disease, symmetrical and continuous, beginning at the rectum and progressing proximally (see Fig. 21.21). The rectum, however, can appear radiologically normal if the patient has been using steroid enemas. Mucosal ulcers, a granular mucosa and thumbprinting are seen, as is blunting of the haustral folds and widening of the presacral space

(>2 cm on a single contrast enema). Inflammatory (pseudo) and filiform (daughter) polyps occur following attacks and in the quiescent phase, respectively. Strictures are rarer than in Crohn's disease and should be differentiated from carcinoma. The incidence of carcinoma rises dramatically in UC if extensive colitis has been present for more than 10 years. Typically patients are invited to enrol in an endoscopic surveillance programme.

The rectum may appear normal on barium enema despite ulcerative colitis being an ascending disease. This is due to the use of steroid enemas.

Infections
Tuberculosis
Colonic tuberculosis (TB) classically affects the terminal ileum. On contrast studies, there is contraction of the caecal wall, upward retraction of the caecum and straightening of the ileocaecal angle. Less than half of cases have pulmonary tuberculosis. TB of the small bowel produces localized areas of thickened, irregular and distorted folds in non-dilated bowel.

Some infections involving the bowel can be conveniently categorized by specific radiological appearances:
- *Colonic 'polyps'*—amoebiasis and schistosomiasis, which usually involve the rectum and can be associated with strictures.
- *Colonic strictures*—schistosomiasis (rectosigmoid); amoebiasis (descending colon); chlamydia, which produces lymphogranuloma venereum (rectosigmoid), is long and tubular, and can undergo malignant change when chronic.
- *Megacolon*—salmonella and amoebiasis.

Angiodysplasia
Angiodysplasia is the result of blood vessel dilatation within the bowel wall, chiefly in the caecum and the ascending colon. This elusive diagnosis, a recognized cause of occult large bowel

bleeding, classically (if rarely) manifests itself angiographically as small pools of contrast with early venous filling. Such angiographic lesions are difficult to confirm by the surgeon or pathologist, but right hemicolectomy is often curative.

Haemorrhoids

A clinical diagnosis. No radiology required. However, this is an important clinical diagnosis to make to avoid unnecessary radiological investigation.

Intestinal obstruction

See Chapter 4.

Pseudomembranous colitis

Pseudomembranous colitis is related to the organism *Clostridium difficile* and antibiotic therapy, particularly clindamycin and third generation cephalosporins. The vast majority of uncomplicated cases are diagnosed by stool culture and treated accordingly without the need for imaging. Plain film features include adynamic bowel, thumbprinting and thickened haustra. The process tends to involve the whole colon. Ascites, small bowel dilatation with oedema of the valvulae conniventes, and thickening and separation of the bowel loops are recognized associations.

Differential diagnoses, radiologically, would include ischaemic colitis and chronic inflammatory bowel disease.

 Barium enema is contraindicated if the bowel is dilated with evidence of thumbprinting on plain film.

Paralytic ileus

See Chapter 4.

Case conferences

Case 1

A 58-year-old lady was admitted to the gastroenterology unit with a 2-month history of diarrhoea. She admits to a 4 kg weight loss over the past 3 months. There were no other symptoms. On clinical and haematological examination she was noted to be anaemic (microcytic hypochromic type). Her CEA was raised at 13.7. There were no other symptoms. Upper GI endoscopy and rigid sigmoidoscopy were normal.

Abdominal radiograph

The bowel gas pattern is normal with no evidence of mechanical obstruction or perforation. No other significant abnormality is seen.

Barium enema

Barium flows freely around the large bowel to the caecum and outlines the appendix. There is a filling defect on the medial wall of the ascending colon which is a constant finding on multiple projections. The appearances are very suspicious of a carcinoma.

Small bowel series

The mucosal pattern of the jejunum and ileum is normal. The terminal ileum outlines normally. There is no evidence of stricturing, ulceration or obstruction.

A colonoscopy was performed and this confirmed a mass lesion in the ascending colon. Multiple biopsies were taken and these confirmed the diagnosis of colonic carcinoma.

CT chest/abdomen/pelvis

A dynamically enhanced multidetector CT study was performed throughout the chest, abdomen and pelvis.

Within the chest, there is no evidence of pulmonary metastases. No hilar or mediastinal lymphadenopathy is seen. On the abdominal images, the liver outlines normally with no evidence of metastases. There is no significant lymphadenopathy or ascites. There is an abnormal mass centred on the ascending colon. The surrounding fat planes are normal. No pelvic lesion is seen.

PET–CT

There is a glucose-avid lesion present within the right colon. The PET–CT location corresponds with that seen on the multidetector CT study. No other areas of increased uptake were identified within the chest, abdomen or pelvis.

A right hemicolectomy was performed. The histological staging was Dukes B.

Case 2
An 82-year-old lady was admitted to hospital with a 3-day history of worsening lower abdominal pain. On examination she was noted to be pyrexial (39.2°C) and had a leucocytosis. She exhibited abdominal tenderness in the suprapubic and left iliac fossa regions. There was no significant past medical history.

Abdominal radiograph
The bowel gas pattern is normal. There is no evidence of intestinal obstruction or perforation.

Ultrasound
The gallbladder, biliary tree, liver, pancreas and spleen outline normally. Both kidneys are sonographically normal. Within the pelvis there is a 6 cm fluid-filled mass seen separately from the bladder. The appearances are very suspicious of an abscess.

Contrast enema
An enema was preformed with water-soluble contrast media. There is significant diverticular disease present with an associated stricture in the sigmoid colon. Scattered diverticula are noted elsewhere. No obstruction or extravasation is seen.

CT abdomen
The upper abdominal viscera are normal. In particular there is no evidence of liver metastases. Within the pelvis, there is a low attenuation mass adjacent to the sigmoid colon. The wall of this is noted to enhance. Sigmoid diverticula are also noted. The appearances are consistent with a pelvic abscess.

CT drainage
(The procedure, including the risks and benefits, were explained. Informed and written consent was obtained. The procedure was performed using an aseptic technique with local analgesia.)

The patient is in the supine position. A skin marker is placed over the site of the collection within the pelvis. The subsequent images demonstrate the local anaesthetic needle in situ. A larger needle is then seen within the collection. A guide wire is placed through the needle and the needle withdrawn. Dilators are passed over the wire into the abscess, a 12F gauge drain is passed over the wire and placed on free drainage.

250 ml of purulent fluid was aspirated and the patient became apyrexial overnight.

Follow-up CT confirmed that the abscess had significantly reduced. It was agreed to resect the diseased strictured segment of sigmoid colon, and a Hartmann's procedure was performed (sigmoid colectomy and oversewing of the rectal stump, with end colostomy). It was anticipated that the colostomy could be reversed in the future and the left colon anastomosed to the rectum when the patient had fully recovered.

7. Scrotal or Groin Mass

The commonest groin masses are hernias and the diagnosis is usually established on clinical examination. Occasionally imaging studies are required to confirm the diagnosis.

Radiological evaluation of the scrotum is usually performed with ultrasound, not only because of the accessible location, but also because of the gonads' radiosensitivity. The most common indication for scrotal ultrasound is to evaluate a mass; the most common diagnosis to exclude is testicular malignancy.

Scrotal mass

Primary testicular neoplasms

Testicular tumours are divided into germ cell and non-germ cell tumours.

Greater than 90% of tumours are germ cell and are typically malignant. Non-germ cell tumours are usually benign. Germ cell tumours are divided into seminomatous and non-seminomatous tumours. The commonest of the latter group is teratoma.

Seminoma

The peak age for presentation of seminoma is the fourth and fifth decades. Although less aggressive than other testicular tumours, metastases are identified at presentation in 25%. On ultrasound, seminoma is characteristically a dark (hypoechoic) solid focal lesion confined within the tunica albuginea (see Fig. 22.19). Calcification and cystic change are rare.

Teratoma

Teratomas tend to be benign in childhood and malignant in adults. On ultrasound, unlike the uniformly hypoechoic seminoma, teratoma is heterogenous with cystic and calcific components.

Secondary malignancy

Lymphoma and leukaemia are the commonest secondary malignancies affecting the testis.

Ultrasound appearances of both are non-specific, although lymphoma is bilateral in half of cases.

Testicular torsion

Testicular torsion is a clinical diagnosis. Although there is no arterial flow within the torted testis, Doppler ultrasound is currently considered unreliable as peripheral and intermittent flow patterns can still be identified in torsion and intermittent torsion, respectively. The diagnosis must therefore be based on the clinical presentation.

Hydrocoele

Hydrocoeles are identified as anechoic (black) areas around the testis (see Fig. 22.18). Septations can be seen on occasion, and indicate chronicity.

The clinical diagnosis of a hydrocoele should be followed up with ultrasound because of the association between hydrocoele and testicular malignancy.

Varicocoele

A varicocoele is a collection of veins around the testis. On Doppler ultrasound, flow can be identified within these vessels, particularly if, while scanning, the patient is asked to increase their intra-abdominal pressure (Valsalva manoeuvre) (see Fig. 22.20). Because the left testicular vein drains into the left renal vein, its obstruction by, for example, a renal cell carcinoma is a recognized association. Therefore, a left-sided varicocoele should prompt inspection of the left kidney to exclude a mass lesion. As the right renal vein drains separately into the IVC, the association does not exist on that side.

Epididymal cysts

The epididymis sits on the posterolateral aspect of the testis, with its head perched on the superior testicular aspect. Cysts are identified as anechoic, echo-free lesions within the epididymal head (see Fig. 22.17). They are a frequent incidental finding in testicular ultrasound and are of no significance. They are not premalignant.

Testicular microlithiasis

Testicular microlithiasis is the presence of myriad tiny calcifications (1–3 mm) within the testis. Their aetiology is obscure. There is some evidence that there is an association with testicular malignancy, so annual surveillance in these patients is currently recommended.

Malignant

Circular and uniform
(may have a necrotic centre)

Benign

Elliptical, fatty centre

Fig. 7.1 Distinguishing the cause of lymphadenopathy.

Inguinal/thigh mass

Hernia

The diagnosis of inguinal hernia is clinical. Unless the hernia contains fluid-filled structures such as small bowel it can be very difficult to appreciate on ultrasound. On occasion, CT or MR is employed when there is diagnostic difficulty. These will show the hernial defect and can identify which structures, if any, are within it. Rarely, herniography—a procedure where contrast is injected directly into the peritoneum, and the patient placed in various positions—is used to outline inguinal hernial sacs. Although this is invasive, it is particularly useful in confirming hernial recurrence.

Saphena varix

Saphena varix is a dilatation of the long saphenous vein, usually at the saphenofemoral junction. It is readily seen on ultrasound, and Doppler ultrasound will show flow and confirm if there is valvular incompetence within the system. It is seen in association with venous insufficiency.

Lymphadenopathy

Lymph nodes are a very common incidental finding on groin ultrasound. They are seen as small, solid, oval masses. As a rule, benign nodes are elliptical and usually have a fatty (bright) centre on ultrasound. Replacement of this by darker, necrotic material—particularly if the nodes are significantly enlarged, circular and matted together—is suspicious of malignant infiltration (Fig. 7.1).

Femoral artery aneurysm

Aneurysms are pathologically enlarged arteries with non-parallel walls. The size, location, presence of flow and thrombus can be determined with ultrasound. Femoral artery aneurysms are rare.

Pseudoaneurysm

This is the name given to abnormal flow and distension within the vessel wall. This is a rare spontaneous event at the groin. However, following interventional procedures such as coronary artery catheterization via a groin puncture, leaking of blood can occur around the artery. This is generally known as a pseudoaneurysm, but is a misnomer. Doppler ultrasound can identify the collection, confirm that there is flow within it and can be used to accurately tamponade the hole. Ultrasound can also be used to guide percutaneous thrombin injection into the collection to thrombose the sac.

Ectopic/undescended testicle

Ultrasound can confirm absence of the testis within the scrotum and can localize testicular material within the inguinal canal. However, it is not effective at locating intra-abdominal testes. CT, and latterly MR, have been employed to identify ectopic testes. MR is preferred because there is no

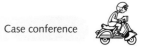

associated radiation (the patient group is generally young) and viable testicular material is bright on T2 weighted sequences (see Part II, Principles of Radiology), making it relatively easy to identify.

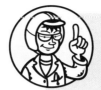 If a femoral aneurysm is detected, look elsewhere for associated abdominal aortic or popliteal aneurysms.

Case conference

A 71-year-old man was admitted to the coronary care unit with severe central chest pain associated with nausea and sweating. ECG demonstrated elevated ST segments in the anterior chest leads consistent with an acute myocardial infarction. Lysis was contraindicated due to a recent haemorrhagic stroke. The decision was made for rescue percutaneous coronary angioplasty (PCA).

The management plan was discussed with the patient as were the risks and benefits of intervention, the patient agreed to coronary stenting if suitable. Coronary angiography confirmed the presence of a high-grade stenosis of the left anterior descending coronary artery. The procedure was technically routine. The following day, it was noted that there was a prominent swelling at the puncture site, with surrounding bruising.

Ultrasound of right groin
The right common, superficial and profunda femoral arteries are identified and are normal. There is good flow in all three vessels. Superficial to the right common femoral vessel there is a cystic collection which measures 1.8 cm. On Doppler imaging, there is active blood flow within it. Furthermore, a jet of blood is seen to emanate from the right common femoral artery into the collection. The appearances are consistent with active extravasation and a 'false aneurysm'.

A trial of compression was undertaken, but repeat ultrasound did not show any interval change. Discussion with the interventional radiologists led to ultrasound-guided percutaneous thrombin injection, which thrombosed the collection successfully.

He was discharged the following week with review arrangements and a number of new medications.

8. Back Pain

Back pain is a very common presenting complaint. The differential diagnosis of the underlying cause is wide, but the commonest cause is mechanical back pain. Classically, plain radiographs have been the mainstay for the imaging of back pain, although it is clear that they are relatively insensitive in excluding significant discovertebral degeneration. MR is the investigation of choice.

Summary of causes
- Degenerative diseases.
- Inflammatory diseases.
- Infection.
- Neoplastic.
- Metabolic.

Degenerative diseases

Disc disease
On the plain lumbar spine radiograph, the characteristic findings of degeneration are narrowing of the intervertebral disc space, sclerosis of the adjacent vertebral bodies and osteophyte formation. On MR imaging, the degenerate, dehydrated disc, unlike the normally hydrated (bright, high signal) disc, appears dark on the T2 weighted (T2W) sequence. This is because it has become dehydrated. Altered signal may be seen in the adjacent vertebral end plates. These zones of altered signal are called 'Modic' changes and help the radiologist determine the chronicity of the degeneration.

It is important to remember that 30% of asymptomatic 30 year olds and almost 100% of 60 year olds will have evidence of disc degeneration on MR. It is crucial therefore to ensure that the radiological findings are consistent with the clinical presentation.

Inflammatory diseases

Seronegative arthropathy
Seronegative arthropathies which affect the vertebral column include psoriasis, enteropathic arthropathies (e.g. ulcerative colitis, Crohn's disease and Whipple's disease), ankylosing spondylitis and Reiter's syndrome (mnemonic: PEAR).

Ankylosing spondylitis
Ankylosing spondylitis primarily affects the axial skeleton (spine, pelvis, hip and shoulder girdle). It typically begins in the sacroiliac joints (see Fig. 23.12b) and goes on to affect the spine. Features on the spinal radiograph include calcification of the annulus fibrosis (syndesmophytes), the 'shiny corner' and 'square vertebra' signs, produced by erosion of the corners of the vertebral bodies and calcification of the anterior longitudinal ligament. Syndesmophytes flowing across several vertebral bodies produce the classical 'bamboo spine' appearance (see Fig. 23.12a).

Enteropathic arthropathy
Conditions such as ulcerative colitis, Crohn's disease and Whipple's disease produce spondylitic changes as in ankylosing spondylitis. The sacroiliac inflammatory changes, as in ankylosing spondylitis, are bilateral and symmetrical.

Psoriatic arthropathy
Like ankylosing spondylitis, the spinal manifestation of this condition is with syndesmophytes and sacroiliitis. The sacroiliitis progresses to bony fusion less commonly than in ankylosing spondylitis, and is unilateral or asymmetrical in just less than half of cases.

Reiter's syndrome
See Chapter 9.

Neoplastic spinal disease

As with neoplasms elsewhere, secondary metastatic deposits are more common than primary bone tumours.

Primary bone tumours
Benign tumours

Benign tumours of the vertebral body include haemangioma, aneurysmal bone cyst, giant cell tumour, osteoid osteoma and osteoblastoma (mnemonic: HAG O2). Osteoblastoma occurs in the posterior elements of the vertebral body and is expansile with a 'soap-bubble' appearance; 50% have calcifications. Osteoid osteoma is usually located within cortical bone and is seen as a sclerotic lesion with a central lucency—the nidus. The classic history is of bone pain, worse at night, and relieved by aspirin.

Malignant tumours
Myeloma and plasmacytoma

On plain films, myeloma looks osteopenic, but has different spinal appearances on CT in its acute and chronic phases. Acutely, there are multiple holes (this has been likened to a 'Swiss cheese'), and chronically trabecular thickening that mimics Paget's disease (see Fig. 23.5). Plasmacytoma is a focal presentation of myeloma. Although it can manifest itself in a variety of ways, the classic appearance on lumbar spine radiograph is of an expansile or destructive lucent lesion. In addition, the appearance of myeloma in the skull is known as 'pepper-pot skull'.

Chordoma

Chordoma is derived from notochordal remnants. 90% of cases occur in two locations, both midline: the clivus (basisphenoid) at the top of the spine, and the sacrum at the bottom. On plain x-rays there is bone destruction and there may be an appreciable soft tissue mass. CT and MR will demonstrate the degree of bone destruction, involvement of adjacent structures and the soft tissue mass.

Secondary bone tumours

On spinal radiographs, metastatic involvement manifests itself as either osteoblastic (bone forming—looks sclerotic; see Fig. 23.11) or osteoclastic (bone resorbing—looks lytic; see Fig. 23.11). Classically, the pedicles are involved and, on the anterior view, this absent pedicle has been likened to an eye winking (the visible 'eye' representing the normal pedicle and the closed eye, the metastatic deposit; Fig. 8.1). Metastatic disease does not generally traverse the intervertebral discs (unlike osteomyelitis, which typically does).

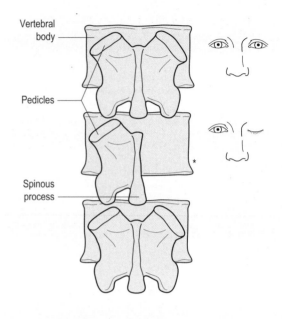

* Absent pedicle on this vertebra

Fig. 8.1 Vertebral spinous metastasis.

It is sometimes possible to suggest the primary location of the cancer by the appearance: sclerotic lesions (bright, bone-forming) occur with prostatic cancer, carcinoid, and lymphoma; lytic disease (dark, bone-losing) is associated with breast and bronchus, and lytic, expansile lesions with the kidney, thyroid, myeloma and melanoma. MRI elegantly demonstrates metastatic disease and also complications such as spinal cord compression (see Fig. 23.14b,c).

Metastatic disease does not generally traverse the intervertebral discs, unlike osteomyelitis.

Metabolic bone disease

Common aetiologies would include:
- Osteoporosis.
- Osteomalacia.
- Rickets.
- Hyperparathyroidism (primary and secondary).
- Acromegaly.

Osteoporosis

Osteoporosis is defined as a reduction of normal quality bone. On spinal x-rays, there is accentuation of the primary (vertical) trabeculae, resorption of the secondary (horizontal) trabeculae and reduced bone density (osteopenia).

These weakened vertebrae are therefore vulnerable and can collapse. This is typically manifest as an anterior wedge fracture or a 'codfish' biconcave collapse. 'Insufficiency' fractures are also seen at the symphysis pubis, femoral neck, pubic rami and sacrum.

The reduction of bone density can be calculated by CT bone density programmes or more usually by dual energy x-ray absorptiometry (DEXA) scan (Fig. 8.2). The score produced measures bone density against healthy bone (T score). A T score between –1.0 and –2.5 represents osteopenia, and less than –2.5, osteoporosis. The 'T' score represents an average score for gender; the 'Z' score is age and gender matched.

In the elderly patient with ongoing hip discomfort following a fall, consider an insufficiency fracture of the pelvis.

Osteomalacia

This is defined as increased uncalcified osteoid in the mature skeleton. Radiographic manifestations include reduction in bone density, coarsening of the trabecular pattern, Looser's zones and bone softening.

Looser's zones (or pseudofractures) represent focal osteoid collections and are seen perpendicular to the long axis of bones. Common sites include the femoral necks, pubic rami and long bones. Bone softening manifests as biconcave vertebral bodies and elsewhere as bowing of the long bones, 'protrusio acetabulae' and basilar invagination of the skull.

Rickets

Rickets is defined as increased uncalcified osteoid in the immature skeleton due to vitamin D deficiency (see Fig. 23.8).

Delayed bone maturation and growth results, but radiographic reduction in bone density is not common. The bone, as in osteomalacia, is softened, and the radiological manifestations generally result from this. In the spine, the vertebrae become biconcave.

Hyperparathyroidism

See Chapter 9.

Acromegaly

Acromegaly is the result of excessive growth hormone's action on the mature skeleton. On plain radiographs, there is an increased sagittal diameter of the chest with an associated kyphosis. The vertebral bodies demonstrate increased anterior and transverse dimensions with 'posterior scalloping' (see also Ch. 9).

Paget's disease

Paget's disease has three phases: lytic, mixed and sclerotic. In the lumbar spine, features include coarsening of the trabeculae and cortices. Pelvic involvement is frequent and coarsening of the iliopectineal line is classic.

Pathological fractures and spinal stenosis may occur. Pelvic Paget's disease may be difficult to discriminate from osteoblastic metastases, but the diagnostic clue is that Paget's disease always begins at a bone end. Metastases occur randomly.

Carefully correlate the pattern of clinical joint disease and bone profile blood results with radiographic appearances.

Isotope bone scans are relatively insensitive to the diagnosis of multiple myeloma because of their lack of osteoblastic activity.

Pelvic Paget's disease can be distinguished from osteoblastic metastases as Paget's disease begins at the bone edge, metastases are random.

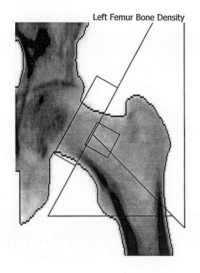

Left Femur Bone Density

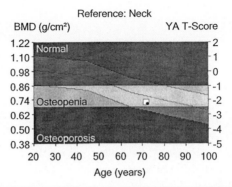

Reference: Neck

Region	BMD [1] (g/cm²)	Young-Adult [2] T-Score	Age-Matched [3] Z-Score
Neck	0.721	-2.2	-0.4
Wards	0.526	-3.0	-0.7
Troch	0.746	-0.4	0.7
Shaft	0.987	-	-
Total	0.832	-1.4	0.1

a

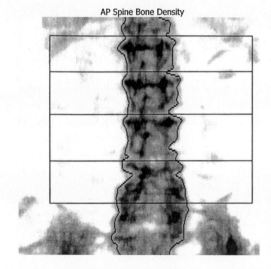

AP Spine Bone Density

Reference: L2-L4

Region	BMD [1] (g/cm²)	Young-Adult [2] T-Score	Age-Matched [3] Z-Score
L1	0.812	-2.7	-0.8
L2	0.814	-3.2	-1.4
L3	0.836	-3.0	-1.2
L4	0.846	-3.0	-1.1
L2-L4	0.833	-3.1	-1.2

b

Fig. 8.2 Bone densitometry results for (a) osteopenic hip, (b) osteoporotic spine.

Case conference

A 48-year-old bricklayer was reviewed at the orthopaedic outpatient clinic. He complained of a 6-week history of severe lower back pain. For the last 2 weeks, the pain had radiated down the left leg to the great toe and was refractory to a number of medications prescribed by the on-call GP service.

On examination his straight leg raising was reduced to 30° on the left, but was normal on the right. The left ankle jerk was also noted to be absent. There was no evidence of any 'red flag' signs.

Lumbar spine radiograph

There is loss of the lumbar lordosis. There is reduction of the L5/S1 disc space with osteophyte formation. There is no evidence of a fracture or vertebral infiltration.

MR lumbar spine

Sagittal T1W, T2W and axial T2W sequences were performed. There is loss of hydration of the lower three lumbar intervertebral disc spaces. There is loss of height of the L5/S1 disc with a posterior disc bulge. On the axial images there is a posterior disc protrusion centrally and towards the left lateral recess. There is significant effacement of the left side of the thecal sac and the prolapsed disc lies adjacent to the left S1 nerve root.

The radiologist informs the orthopaedic registrar at ward level who arranges a clinically suitable date for surgery.

9. Joint Pain

Joint pain causes significant physical and functional burden. Despite great technical strides in nuclear medicine, ultrasound, CT and MRI, plain radiographs remain the mainstay of clinical imaging.

Frequently plain radiographs are requested initially, but the yield of significant findings may be limited in relation to clinical symptoms. Further imaging should be tailored to the most likely diagnoses:

- Rheumatoid arthritis.
- Seronegative arthritis.
- Degenerative.
- Haemophilia.
- Metabolic.
- Infectious.
- Systemic.

Rheumatoid arthritis

Rheumatoid arthritis (RA) is a multisystem autoimmune disorder, where a symmetrical synovial and cartilaginous joint pathology is a variable component of systemic disease. The appendicular joints affected include those of the hands, feet, wrists, knees, ankles, elbows, hips and shoulders. The axial skeleton may also be affected, i.e. the atlantoaxial and apophyseal joints.

The hand
On hand radiographs, RA tends to affect the metacarpophalangeal (MCP), proximal interphalangeal (PIP) and the intercarpal joints. In the wrist, the ulnar styloid and distal radioulnar joints are affected. The disease tends to affect the proximal portion of the joint surface more severely than the distal (see Fig. 23.21).

Initially there are joint effusions with synovial thickening, periarticular oedema and osteoporosis. The changes are symmetrical. This is followed by joint space narrowing and erosion at the joint margins. In complicated cases, subluxation and malalignment of joints is seen with ulnar deviation, swan-neck and boutonnière deformity of the fingers, and ankylosis (fusion).

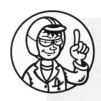
Rheumatoid arthritis affects the MCP and PIP joints; osteoarthritis typically affects the distal interphalangeal (DIP) joints.

Atlantoaxial joint
The cervical region of the spine is most commonly affected. Pathological change in the transverse atlantoaxial ligament (either laxity or ligament rupture) produces subluxation of the joint (Fig. 9.1). In 25% of severe RA patients, atlantoaxial subluxation can be demonstrated on flexion and extension lateral cervical spine radiographs. The distance between the posterior aspect of the anterior arch of the atlas and the dens should not exceed 3 mm in the adult. A wider space or one which changes between flexion and extension indicates subluxation. Radiographs of the atlantoaxial joint may also show erosions of the odontoid peg. Subluxation may affect other cervical levels, particularly C4/C5.

The hip and knee
The characteristic differentiation between rheumatoid and osteoarthritis (OA) at these joints is the uniform reduction in joint space seen in RA. OA has a more asymmetrical joint space involvement, affecting the superior aspect of the acetabular joint space at the hip and the medial compartment space of the knee. OA also tends to have more periarticular sclerotic change.

Seronegative arthritis

Psoriasis
Psoriatic arthropathy occurs in 5% of patients with psoriasis. The relationship with skin disease is variable. There are several arthropathic patterns in psoriasis: the commonest is single joint involvement; others include a rheumatoid arthritis type appearance, an arthritis affecting the DIP

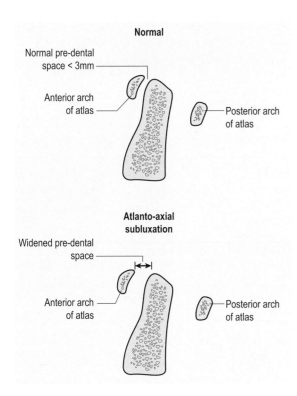

Normal

Normal pre-dental space < 3mm

Anterior arch of atlas

Posterior arch of atlas

Atlanto-axial subluxation

Widened pre-dental space

Anterior arch of atlas

Posterior arch of atlas

Fig. 9.1 Atlanto-axial subluxation (lateral projection).

joints, a spinal distribution and finally an arthritis mutilans.

Types of psoriatic arthropathy include:
- Mono/oligoarthritis.
- Ankylosing spondylitis.
- DIP predominance.
- Arthritis mutilans.
- Rheumatoid distribution.

Hands and feet
Soft tissue swelling is prominent, and involvement of a whole finger is known as a dactylitis ('sausage digit'). The arthropathy, which is asymmetric, is destructive and affects the DIP joints, with erosions beginning peripherally at the joint margins and advancing centrally ('cup and pencil' deformity). Tuft resorption may also be seen (see Fig. 23.17). A fine 'whiskering' can also be seen at the attachments of ligaments and tendons (the entheses). Bone density is normal.

Spine and sacroiliac joints
The sacroiliac changes are similar to those of ankylosing spondylitis, being symmetrical and bilateral. The spinal appearances (spondylitis),

however, are characteristically asymmetrical. Paravertebral ossification is a characteristic feature. Any spinal level may be affected.

Reiter's syndrome
This predominantly male disease is usually the sequela of sexually transmitted disease or dysentery and describes the association of urethritis, arthritis, eye and skin lesions. The arthropathy of Reiter's syndrome affects the feet and hands, the spine and the sacroiliac (SI) joints. X-ray appearances in the hands and feet are similar to psoriasis, with the foot more commonly affected than the hand. Calcaneal 'spurs' are a feature. SI joint appearances are similar to ankylosing spondylitis and psoriasis, with the spondylitic changes indistinguishable from psoriasis.

Ankylosing spondylitis
Ankylosing spondylitis usually affects young people. The disease, although it may affect large and even small joints, typically presents in the spine and sacroiliac joints. The presence of extra-axial disease is important as it alters clinical management (see Ch. 8).

Enteropathy
Patients with ulcerative colitis, Crohn's disease and Whipple's disease can suffer from spinal and sacroiliac arthropathies similar to those seen in ankylosing spondylitis. Peripheral joint involvement is rarer, and features include loss of bone density, soft tissue swelling and synovitis. These changes reflect exacerbations of the disease—the peripheral arthropathy resolves as the disease remits, the spinal pathology does not.

Degeneration

Osteoarthritis
Osteoarthritis may be primary (polyarticular) or secondary (monoarticular). In the hands, the first carpal, metacarpal and intercarpal joints are affected. In the feet the first metatarsophalangeal joint is affected. Osteophytes, sclerosis and geodes (subchondral cysts) are characteristic, as is non-uniform joint narrowing and an asymmetrical distribution (see Figs 23.15, 23.23, 23.24; see also Ch. 8).

Radiographic features of osteoarthritis are illustrated in Figure 9.2.

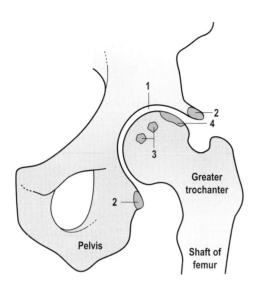

Fig. 9.2 Osteoarthritic changes at the hip: 1. Narrowed joint space; 2. osteophytes; 3. bone cysts; 4. subchondral sclerosis.

gout usually affects only one joint—often the first metatarsophalangeal joint of the foot (podagra). This manifests as soft tissue swelling, joint effusions and loss of bone density around the joint. Chronically (chronic tophaceous gout), non-calcified nodules of calcium urate (tophi) adjacent to the joint are identified. Erosions, round or oval, lie in the long axis of the bone, pointing away from the joint (see Fig. 23.13). Intraosseous tophi—small cysts within the bone—are also seen. Bone density is normal. Diagnosis is by detection of negatively birefringent crystals from a joint aspirate.

With an acute, red, hot, painful, swollen joint, septic arthritis should be excluded by joint aspiration.

Haemophilia

Haemosiderin from a haemarthrosis is absorbed by synovium which consequently becomes enlarged and prone to injury. This injury causes bleeding, more haemosiderin production and further synovial enlargement. Haemorrhage also produces articular cartilage changes.

Radiographic features include joint effusions and epiphyseal enlargement secondary to hyperaemic osteopenia. In the knee, there is epiphyseal enlargement, widening of the intercondylar notch and squaring of the inferior aspect of the patella. Subchondral cysts and joint space narrowing are also seen. At the ankle joint, tibiotalar slant is seen, secondary to narrowing of the lateral aspect of the distal tibial epiphysis. The 'haemophilic pseudotumour' may be seen in the pelvis. This manifests as an expansile lucent area within bone, usually the ilium.

Metabolic disorders

Gout
Gout results from hyperuricaemia and presents with recurrent acute arthritis. In the acute phase,

Calcium pyrophosphate dehydrate (CPPD) deposition disease
CPPD is the commonest cause of an acutely swollen joint in the over 60-year-old age group.

CPPD deposition disease is the association of pseudogout, chondrocalcinosis and an arthropathy. Pseudogout indicates a crystal synovitis that causes an acute inflammatory arthritis. Radiological findings in pseudogout are of joint effusions and soft tissue oedema. Chondrocalcinosis is not a specific disease, but a radiological sign meaning the identification of joint crystals on x-ray. These can be CPPD or hydroxyapatite crystals. Hydroxyapatite crystal deposition is associated with hyperparathyroidism and milk–alkali syndrome.

In chronic CPPD arthropathy, features include subchondral cysts, articular surface breakdown and intra-articular fragments. Typical sites include the patellofemoral, elbow, radiocarpal and MCP joints. Chondrocalcinosis, if present, tends to be seen in large joints like the shoulder, the hip and the knee. The destructive arthropathy can mimic neuropathic joints (a pseudoneuropathy), but neurological examination is normal.

49

Gout (uric acid) and pseudogout (CPPD) can be distinguished by the birefringence pattern of the crystals in the aspirated joint fluid.

Haemochromatosis

The arthropathy in haemochromatosis is due to the deposition of iron in the articular cartilage. Radiologically, the changes resemble CPPD with a predilection for the MCP joints of the second and third metacarpals, the midcarpals and the carpometacarpal joints, with beak or hook-like osteophytes. Chondrocalcinosis is frequent.

Infectious diseases

Osteomyelitis

Conventional radiographs are relatively insensitive in osteomyelitis. Up to 50% of bone has to be resorbed before bone destruction is visible, and x-ray changes can lag significantly behind clinical findings. Radiographic findings include soft tissue swelling, periosteal reaction, osteoporosis, reactive sclerosis, sequestrum, involucrum, soft tissue abscesses and sinus tract formation. Bone scans are positive within hours of the onset of symptoms. A focal hotspot is the most common finding. On MRI the inflammation is seen to cause decreased signal on T1 weighted (T1W) and increased signal on T2W sequences. Good delineation of the extent of the disease—especially bone marrow, periosteal and surrounding soft tissue structures—is possible. MRI is more sensitive in the acute/subacute than the chronic phase.

Brodie's abscess (subacute osteomyelitis)

This describes a local bone infection, usually seen before epiphyseal closure, in the tibial or femoral metaphysis. *Staphylococcus aureus* is the usual causative organism. On plain x-rays, this is seen as a well-defined lucent lesion at the end of a long bone. There may be marginal sclerosis or periosteal reaction.

Systemic diseases

Hypertrophic pulmonary osteoarthropathy (HPOA)

HPOA describes specific bony manifestations seen in a variety of systemic illnesses. These manifestations include a laminated periosteal reaction which affects the distal radius, ulna, tibia and fibula. It is associated with finger clubbing and the aetiology is given by the mnemonic 'CLUBBING':

C   Cyanotic heart disease
L   Liver cirrhosis
U   Ulcerative colitis and Crohn's disease
B   Bronchiectasis (and other purulent lung disease such as empyema and abscess)
B   Bacterial endocarditis
I   Idiopathic
NG   New growth (neoplasm).

A 37-year-old medical secretary presents with a 6-month history of discomfort in the small joints of the hands. In particular she had found it especially troublesome removing her rings. She has a past medical history of pernicious anaemia, diagnosed 10 years ago. The joints were particularly stiff in the mornings but improve after 2 hours of use. On examination there was evidence of active synovitis at the MCP and PIP joints.

She was commenced on non-steroidal anti-inflammatory drugs (NSAIDs) with good effect while awaiting results of blood tests and radiographs of the hands.

Radiograph of hands
The bones are osteopenic. There are erosive changes bilaterally at the MCP and PIP joints. Ulnar deviation of the phalanges is noted. The appearances are consistent with rheumatoid arthritis.

She was commenced on methotrexate, 10 mg weekly. Over the following 7 years she tried several disease-modifying anti-rheumatic drugs (DMARDs) with variable benefit before starting adalimumab therapy. At routine review she complained of increasing dyspnoea and a dry cough.

Chest radiograph
The cardiac contour and pulmonary vascularity are normal. There are reticulonodular shadows present in both lungs, chiefly in the mid and lower zones. No focal mass lesion is evident. The appearances are consistent with interstitial lung disease.

Pulmonary function tests demonstrated a restrictive abnormality and a transfer factor of 48%. High resolution CT was performed.

High resolution CT of the chest
There are subpleural interstitial changes present in both lungs, chiefly in the lower zones. No focal mass is identified. There is no endobronchial mass or significant lymphadenopathy. The appearances are consistent with a linear non-septal pattern of interstitial lung disease. The history of methotrexate therapy and rheumatoid arthritis is noted, and the appearances would be in keeping with either of these. The differential diagnosis for these appearances would include amiodarone therapy, fibrosing alveolitis, asbestos-related lung disease and other connective tissue diseases.

Her rheumatologist discontinued her methotrexate and made arrangements for follow up under the care of the respiratory physicians.

Neck masses have been historically divided into midline, anterior and posterior triangle masses. Latterly, anatomical localization by disease level (the Sloane–Kettering Level I–VI classification) has gained widespread acceptance among head and neck surgeons. Ultrasound is very valuable for the evaluation of neck masses due to their relatively superficial location. Biopsy of the mass can be undertaken at this stage. Further characterization and staging is performed with a combination of CT, MR and PET scanning.

Summary of causes

- Thyroid masses.
- Salivary diseases.
- Lymphadenopathy.
- Congenital/developmental.
- Miscellaneous.

Thyroid masses

Single nodule

Approximately 5% of the adult population have a thyroid nodule. Greater than 85–90% of thyroid nodules are benign and, if less than 1.5 cm in size, are likely to be occult (i.e. an incidental imaging finding).

A single nodule is the commonest nodular disease of the thyroid (80% of cases). Cystic change occurs in the majority of individuals (see Fig. 24.22). The presence of solid masses within the cyst, a size greater than 1 cm or the presence of microcalcification merits fine needle aspiration (FNA) to exclude cystic papillary carcinoma.

Indications for FNA of a thyroid nodule include:
- Solid mass within the cyst.
- Size >1 cm.
- Microcalcification.

Adenomas

These account for 10% of thyroid nodular disease and are focal gland proliferations. They have a capsule which is demonstrated as the 'halo' sign on ultrasound. The distinction between follicular adenoma and carcinoma requires histology, but the demonstration of follicular cells on cytology represents an indication for surgical resection. When follicular neoplasms are resected, 80% are benign and 20% malignant.

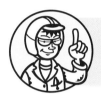

Evidence of papillary cells is strongly correlated with malignancy.

Hyperfunctioning nodules

These may be hyperplastic or adenomas and have no specific sonographic characteristics.

Papillary carcinoma

This is the commonest malignancy of the thyroid gland, accounting for two-thirds of thyroid malignancy. On ultrasound, these are seen as hypoechoic masses with a surrounding capsule. Microcalcifications are often present. The tumour is hypervascular on Doppler US. Fifty percent of patients have local nodal involvement at presentation. The finding of papillary cells on FNA is strongly correlated with malignancy as in practice they rarely represent an adenoma. The surgical procedure of choice, when papillary carcinoma is diagnosed, is total thyroidectomy.

Follicular carcinoma

This accounts for 20% of thyroid carcinomas and is associated with hyperplastic or adenomatous nodules in two-thirds of cases. There are no specific sonographic features but a thickened capsule and 'chaotic' vessels on Doppler ultrasound are described. The finding of follicular cells on FNA is an indication for surgery. Eighty percent of cases are benign and 20% malignant. The surgical procedure of choice for a follicular mass is a hemithyroidectomy, with resection of the affected lobe and the isthmus. If malignant, completion thyroidectomy should be considered.

Anaplastic carcinoma

On ultrasound, this is hypoechoic, with areas of necrosis, amorphous calcification and local invasion. Anaplastic carcinoma has the worst prognosis. Overall, the most accurate sign of malignancy on ultrasound is microcalcification.

For the role of nuclear medicine in the thyroid nodule and in the parathyroid, see Part II.

Salivary diseases

Parotid adenoma

Parotid adenoma (also known as pleomorphic adenoma or benign mixed tumour of the parotid) is the commonest mass of the parotid space (80%), occurring more commonly in females than in males, typically in the age range 30–60 years. The CT/MR appearances are those of a well-circumscribed, mildly enhancing mass (see Fig. 24.23). Cross-sectional imaging allows delineation of the mass relative to the facial nerve (i.e. within the superficial or deep lobe of the parotid).

Warthin's tumour (adenolymphoma)

This benign tumour is more commonly seen in males (>60 years) and has a strong association with smoking. The tumour occurs typically in the parotid tail. It is usually inhomogeneous on CT/MR, with cystic areas and foci of haemorrhage. Mild contrast enhancement occurs. There is also increased uptake of fluorodeoxyglucose on PET scanning.

Parotid carcinoma

There are two tumour types: mucoepidermoid (60%) and adenoid cystic carcinoma. The role of cross-sectional imaging is to:
1. Confirm that the lesion is within the parotid.
2. Locate it either within the deep or the superficial lobe.

Radiologically, parotid carcinoma is an invasive intraparotid mass which enhances with contrast. Clinically, the mass is painful, and an association with facial nerve palsy is characteristic.

Sjögren's syndrome

Sjögren's syndrome is a chronic autoimmune disease which may be primary or secondary. Destruction of the lacrimal glands is a recognized feature. The imaging findings will depend on the stage of the disease. In the early stages on cross-sectional imaging, there are bilateral small cystic areas. Later, there are larger cysts (see Fig. 24.24) and solid lymphocytic masses with parenchymal destruction. Punctate calcification is also a feature. Sjögren's syndrome can be complicated by non-Hodgkin's lymphoma.

Lymphadenopathy

The most important question in the clinical imaging of lymph nodes is to separate reactive (benign) nodes from metastatic malignant nodes. This can prove challenging. Size is not an absolute criterion, but neck nodes greater than 1.5 cm are viewed with suspicion. In addition, persistent nodes identified in the posterior triangle of the neck represent cause for concern. Benign nodes tend to be elliptical, whereas malignant nodes are circular. The fatty centre of benign nodes is replaced by hypoechoic necrotic tissue in malignancy. PET scanning is playing an increasing clinical role in determining reactive from malignant cervical lymphadenopathy.

Congenital/developmental diseases

Thyroglossal (duct) cyst

Thyroglossal duct cyst is the commonest congenital neck lesion. It arises from the thyroglossal duct, which lies between the tongue's foramen caecum (superiorly) and the thyroid bed (inferiorly). It is classically a painless, mobile, midline swelling, but the site can be more lateral, inferiorly. It usually presents in the first decade, although 10% are seen in the third and fourth decades.

On ultrasound, it is anechoic. CT demonstrates a low attenuation mass and, on MRI, cystic composition (low signal T1 weighted, high signal T2 weighted).

The presence of a solid mass or calcification should raise suspicion of a complicating papillary carcinoma of the thyroid (rare, less than 1%).

Branchial cyst

This cyst develops from the second branchial cleft and occurs in teenagers and young adults. Branchial cysts are significantly more common in males. The commonest of branchial anomalies (95%), it presents as a mass at the anterior aspect of the sternomastoid muscle, typically the upper third. On ultrasound, CT and MR it is cystic with non-enhancing walls unless infected. It contains variable quantities of protein which produce a spectrum of signals on MR imaging.

Cystic hygroma

Cystic hygroma (also known as lymphangioma) is composed of dilated lymphatic spaces, usually presents at birth and early childhood, and has an association with Turner's syndrome. It is multiloculated and characteristically insinuates itself between neck structures, but without any significant mass effect. On ultrasound, CT and MR the appearances are those of a cystic lesion. Haemorrhage may be present within the lesion.

Miscellaneous disorders

Carotid body tumour

Carotid body tumour (also known as chemodectoma, paraganglionoma) is a tumour of the glomus body (paraganglia). On angiography, there is characteristic splaying of the internal and carotid arteries (the 'inverted stirrup' sign) and a 'blush' by the tumour. CT demonstrates a markedly enhancing mass (see Fig. 24.25). On MR imaging there is, on T1 weighted sequences, a 'salt and pepper' appearance—the 'salt' representing haemorrhage, and the 'pepper' signal, flow void. The condition may be sporadic or familial (autosomal dominant).

Laryngocoele

A laryngocoele is an acquired saccular swelling sited lateral to the thyrohyoid membrane and represents herniation of respiratory epithelium through a membrane defect. It can be identified on plain x-rays as an air shadow lateral to the larynx. CT will confirm the relationship to the thyrohyoid membrane.

Pharyngeal pouch

Pharyngeal pouch occurs between the two bands of the inferior constrictor muscle (Killian's dehiscence). The presentation is typically with the regurgitation of undigested food or occasionally with a neck lump in those over 50 years of age. Barium swallow appearances demonstrate filling of a pouch at the level of the lower cervical vertebrae (see Ch. 3).

Lipoma and sebaceous cyst

These two superficial lesions should be readily differentiated by ultrasound. A lipoma has echogenic characteristics which should be identical to the surrounding fatty tissues. A sebaceous cyst tends to be more hypoechoic and of a fluid nature. They also have characteristic appearances on MRI (see Fig. 24.26).

Fine needle aspiration cytology (FNAC) is the gold standard investigation for a neck mass.

Case conference

A 28-year-old lady was referred by her general practitioner to surgical outpatients with a right-sided neck mass. On examination, there was a firm swelling below and lateral to the right of the thyroid cartilage. No other abnormality was evident. She had no overt clinical features of thyroid disease.

Ultrasound of neck
A well-defined 1.8 × 2.3 cm hypoechoic mass is identified in the right lobe of the thyroid. The mass is well encapsulated and predominantly solid, with some cystic spaces. Small areas of calcification are also noted. The remainder of the thyroid outlines normally. There is no significant lymphadenopathy. A subsequent isotope scan demonstrated a corresponding photopenic region within the right lobe. The appearances were felt to be consistent with a 'cold nodule'. Thyroid function tests were also normal.

Ultrasound-guided FNA
The procedure was explained, as were the risks, benefits and complications. Written and informed consent was obtained. Using an aseptic technique, a 21 gauge needle was advanced into the lesion under ultrasound control. Cells were aspirated, spread onto slides and sent to the cytology department.

A population of follicular cells was identified, and on this basis the patient was referred for thyroid surgery. The final histology was that of a follicular adenoma.

Conclusion
A hemithyroidectomy was performed. The patient's postoperative course was routine and she was discharged.

11. Neurological Symptoms

Neurological pathologies account for a significant proportion of hospital morbidity and mortality. Prompt medical and surgical management with appropriate imaging are crucial.

Unlike most other body systems, the plain film has only very limited application in neuroimaging. Its role is restricted to traumatic head injury and even then is of limited benefit. The mainstay of neuroimaging is computed tomography (CT), especially for trauma and suspected subarachnoid haemorrhage, and magnetic resonance imaging (MRI). The radiologist has an increasing role in the treatment of cerebral aneurysms by 'coiling' procedures.

Headache

Headache is a common complaint and is usually benign in nature. The vast majority of patients require no investigations; however, a detailed history is crucial as there are several 'red flags' (signs) that suggest potentially serious causes of headache.

Core symptoms prompting early radiological investigations

Sudden, severe headache

This is particularly relevant if found in association with nausea, vomiting and neck stiffness. In this circumstance it is mandatory that subarachnoid haemorrhage (SAH) is excluded. Patients will often describe the headache as 'the worst of my life' and 'I thought I was going to die'. The investigation of choice is cranial CT.

SAH is confirmed by the presence of hyperdensity in the subarachnoid spaces (see Fig. 24.13). The patient requires additional imaging to visualize the intracranial vessels as, in 85% of such cases, the cause is a ruptured intracranial aneurysm. In 5% of cases, a ruptured arteriovenous malformation is the source and in 10% of patients no treatable cause is found. CT angiography (CTA) has replaced invasive catheter angiography in many centres (see Fig. 24.14), with catheter angiography reserved for inconclusive cases (see Fig. 24.7).

Headache worse in the mornings and/or on standing

Particularly in association with nausea and vomiting, this is suggestive of raised intracranial pressure (ICP) and is often due the development of hydrocephalus. This is an increase in pressure within the ventricular system, due either to an obstruction of the cerebrospinal fluid (CSF) pathway or overproduction of CSF. Although initial investigation is usually CT, MRI is the investigation of choice. Obstruction to CSF flow can be produced by tumours or cysts, especially in the midline, involving the third or fourth ventricle.

On CT, the ventricles are seen to be dilated (see Fig. 24.18a), the earliest changes being seen in the temporal horns of the lateral ventricles.

A colloid cyst in the base of the septum pellucidum often obstructs the outflow from both lateral ventricles at the level of the foramina of Monroe (see Fig. 24.18). It can present with postural headaches and is a recognized cause of sudden death. On CT it is a low attenuation lesion seen at the foramen of Monroe. Signal characteristics are variable on MR depending on the protein content. There is no contrast enhancement on CT or MR.

In children, posterior fossa tumours are more common than supratentorial lesions and often present with hydrocephalus due to obstruction of the fourth ventricle (see Fig. 24.16). Excessive CSF production results in a non-obstructive (or communicating) hydrocephalus. Figure 24.15 demonstrates a lateral ventricular papilloma in a child, presenting with lethargy and sunset eyes. The latter is a classic finding in children with hydrocephalus.

Focal neurological deficit

Acute presentation

The presentation of a focal neurological deficit that is sudden and heralded as a unilateral limb weakness (hemiparesis) with or without speech difficulties (dysphasia) indicates a cerebrovascular accident (CVA) or stroke.

CT performed early after onset (less than 3 hours) is often normal, although early signs of infarction may be appreciated (see Fig. 24.17). Its primary role, however, is in detecting haemorrhagic transformation that would preclude antiplatelet or anticoagulant treatment. CT will also identify those patients with a large intracerebral haemorrhage (see Fig. 24.19). These present in a similar fashion but usually have significantly altered consciousness (decreased Glasgow Coma Scale) and/or a history of severe headache at onset.

Those haemorrhages centred on the basal ganglia and in the deep cerebellar hemisphere white matter are usually due to underlying hypertension. The hypertension produces arteriosclerotic changes in the perforator vessels supplying these territories which results in a weakening within the vessel wall and a propensity to rupture. Other causes of intracerebral haemorrhage should also be considered.

Ruptured intracranial aneurysms can result in predominant intracerebral haematoma rather than subarachnoid haemorrhage (see Fig. 24.19). This classically occurs with middle cerebral artery aneurysms which rupture into the Sylvian fissure. Haemorrhage into pre-existing tumours may also occur.

Subacute presentation

A history of increasing neurological deficit over a period of time is more typical of a growing mass lesion, e.g. meningioma. The length of history reflects the nature of the underlying mass, with malignant tumours presenting within weeks, but more benign lesions over a period of months.

Cross-sectional imaging will identify and measure the dimensions of the mass. The location may be important in the differential diagnosis, e.g. sphenoidal ridge cerebellopontine angle (see Fig. 24.21). Characteristics of the mass may also provide further aetiological clues: a mural nodule within the mass (cystic astrocytoma); calcification or dural tail (meningioma, see Fig. 24.20); cystic degeneration and necrosis (glioblastoma multiforme) or crossing the midline (butterfly glioma).

A group known generically as a 'white matter diseases' is the most common inflammatory disorder of the CNS. The most prevalent in the western world is multiple sclerosis, characterized by destruction of normally formed myelin, with relative axonal preservation. The aetiology is unknown. Most patients present in the third or fourth decade. The first clinical symptom is often impaired or double vision (diplopia). Other common symptoms include weakness, tingling, numbness and gait disturbances. With disease progression, loss of sphincter control, blindness, paralysis and dementia may develop.

The diagnosis is fundamentally a clinical one; however, MRI sensitivity exceeds clinical examination alone as well as all other imaging modalities including CT. The diagnosis is usually made with reference to the clinical, laboratory and imaging findings.

Multiple sclerosis is a clinical diagnosis supported by MRI findings.

MRI features include high signal on T2 weighted sequences in the periventricular white matter, often characteristically oval in shape ('Dawson's fingers'). These may be best appreciated in the sagittal images. Other common locations for demyelinating plaques are the corpus callosum and the craniocervical junction of the cord (classically C2 level; see Fig. 24.12).

Seizures

A seizure is the result of an abnormal electrical discharge within the brain. Epilepsy is a condition characterized by more than one seizure. The role of neuroimaging is to identify a structural epileptogenic focus. Symptomatic seizures may be acute due to a precipitant or remote to a pre-existent lesion, with seizure the main or only symptom. In adults acute symptomatic seizures are most commonly caused by trauma (see Fig. 24.10), cerebrovascular disease, tumours (see Fig. 24.3), drug withdrawal (including alcohol), CNS infection and degenerative disease. In children with seizures, a metabolic disease should also be considered.

Remote seizures are caused by previous trauma, CVA, CNS infection, tumour, atrophy, malformations of cortical development and hippocampal sclerosis (see Fig. 24.4).

Most of these causes are identifiable with CT or MRI, with the latter providing the better yield. For acute symptomatic seizure, CT is recommended. MRI should be arranged for non-acute symptomatic seizures with confusion and postictal deficit. In a child with unexplained cognitive or motor delays and less than 1 year of age, MRI is recommended. All patients with partial seizures, abnormal electroencephalograms (EEGs) and generalized epilepsy should also be imaged.

 The nature of the seizure may indicate the location of a structural focus.

Head trauma

Trauma is the most common cause of death and permanent disability in the first few decades of life, with head trauma the main culprit. The annual incidence of head injury is 0.2–0.3% per year, peaking at ages 15–24 years where the incidence is 500–600 per 100,000 population. The incidence declines until the sixth decade when it increases again. Up to 10% of head injuries are fatal, with 20–40% of moderate severity. Males are affected four times more commonly than females. In the second and third decades, road traffic accidents (RTAs) and assaults account for the majority. Falls are the most common cause at the extremes of age. Two-thirds of head injury mortality occurs before hospitalization.

The principal imaging test in neurotrauma is CT, usually without contrast enhancement (non contrast CT). MRI has a limited role acutely. Clinical severity is assessed using the Glasgow Coma Scale (GCS). In mild head injury (GCS 13–15), observation is often all that is required. CT is reserved for those patients with persistent headache and/or vomiting. All patients with moderate (GCS 8–12) and severe (GCS less than 8) injury require imaging to detect haematomas requiring surgical intervention. The full extent of brain injury will not be completely determined with CT alone. Although MRI provides more accurate information regarding the prognosis, limited availability, in particular within the UK, limits its use.

Head injuries incurred can be classified into two groups:
- Primary lesions.
- Secondary lesions.

Primary lesions
Primary lesions are due to direct neuronal injury, primary haemorrhage and primary vascular injuries.

Primary neuronal
Nearly all primary neuronal injuries occur following shear-strain deformation by rotational acceleration of the head. Characteristic locations include diffuse axonal injuries (see Fig. 24.10b), cortical contusions, subcortical grey matter injury and brain stem injury (see Fig. 24.10a). The sensitivity of CT in detecting these is low compared with MRI.

Primary haemorrhage
Primary haemorrhage results from injury to any of the cerebral vessels (meningeal, pial, artery, vein, capillary). The type of haemorrhage is dependent on the vessel injured.

Extradural haematoma
Extradural haematoma (EDH) is usually arterial and caused by direct laceration or tearing of meningeal arteries (often the middle meningeal artery) by skull fracture; these are often temporal or temporoparietal in location. Venous EDH is less common and results from laceration of a dural sinus by the fracture; these are usually in the posterior fossa.

On NCCT images, the EDH is identified as a biconvex ('lens shaped') area of high attenuation adjacent to the skull (see Fig. 24.11). An underlying fracture may be appreciated on the bony windows.

Subdural haematoma
Subdural haematoma (SDH) is typically caused by stretching and tearing of bridging veins that traverse the subdural space. The symptoms of an isolated SDH vary from asymptomatic to unconsciousness. The outcome is often poor due to secondary injuries and associated additional injuries.

On NCCT images, the SDH is identified as a crescentic mass adjacent to the skull bone (Fig. 11.1; see also Fig. 24.8). As a rule, acute SDH

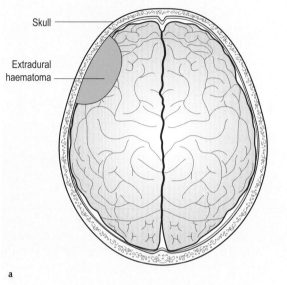

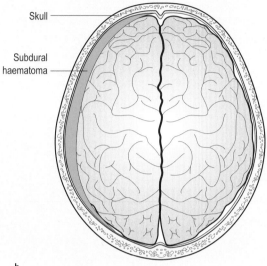

Fig. 11.1 Extradural (a) and subdural haematoma (b).

(within 2 weeks) is of higher attenuation than the brain, subacute SDH (2–4 weeks) isoattenuating with the brain, and chronic SDH (greater than 4 weeks) of lower attenuation than the brain.

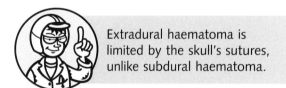

Extradural haematoma is limited by the skull's sutures, unlike subdural haematoma.

Intracerebral haematoma

Intracerebral haematoma (ICH) most commonly arises from rotational shear/strain injury to intraparenchymal arteries or veins. Occasionally direct penetrating injury to the vessel is the cause. Haematoma size varies from millimetres to several centimetres. ICH is usually within the frontal temporal white matter or basal ganglia.

On NCCT, these are high attenuation lesions with mass effect. If large, effacement of the ventricles and midline shift may be appreciated. It is important to look for 'contra-coup' injuries: with a frontal haematoma, review the occipital region for small petechial areas of high attenuation.

Intraventricular haemorrhage

Intraventricular haemorrhage (IVH) is quite common and can be caused by a variety of traumatic lesions, e.g. diffuse axonal injury (DAI), intracranial haemorrhage (ICH) and large contusions. It is most commonly due to tearing of subependymal veins within the ventricular walls. Traumatic SAH can also occur.

On NCCT there are high attenuation areas with fluid levels in the ventricles. The most common location is the occipital horns of the lateral ventricles.

Primary vascular

Primary vascular injuries include caroticocavernous fistulae (see Fig. 24.5), arterial dissections/occlusions, dural sinus lacerations and occlusions. There is often a significant delay from trauma to onset of symptoms. Those that are symptomatic are often unrecognized as they are masked by other intra- or extracranial injuries. Patients with basal skull fractures are particularly at risk (see Fig. 24.9).

Secondary effects of traumatic brain injury include arterial infarction, diffuse hypoxic injury (see Fig. 24.6), diffuse brain swelling/oedema and pressure necrosis from brain displacement and herniation.

Case conference

A 42-year-old lady was admitted to A&E following collapse and loss of consciousness. Her husband, who had been at home with her, said that she had complained of a very severe headache for a short time prior to her collapse.

CT brain
On the unenhanced scan, there is hyperdensity in the subarachnoid spaces, most prominent in the right Sylvian fissure and the cisterna ambiens. There is no evidence of a mass lesion or midline shift. The appearances are consistent with subarachnoid haemorrhage.

A CT angiogram performed at the same time demonstrates a saccular enhancing lesion arising from the supraclinoid portion of the right internal carotid artery at the origin of the right posterior communicating (PCom) artery. The appearances are in keeping with a right PCom aneurysm.

After discussion with the neurosurgeons, it was agreed that endovascular occlusion was the preferred therapeutic option. The procedure was fully explained to the patient and her husband, together with the risks, benefits and alternatives. Written and informed consent was obtained.

Endovascular occlusion
The patient underwent general anaesthesia in the neurointerventional suite. A right femoral sheath was placed via Seldinger technique. Once full systemic heparinization was instituted, a guiding catheter was placed in the distal cervical right internal carotid artery. A coaxial catheter was advanced, through the guiding catheter, into the aneurysm sac at the level of the right PCom artery. Five detachable coils were deployed within the sac. The procedure was technically routine, with no complications recorded.

The patient was returned to the neurosurgical unit. Hydration was maintained (3 L in 24 hours). Close observations were instituted to check for evidence of stroke or hydrocephalus. The patient made a full neurological recovery.

Arrangements will be made for follow-up for a postcoiling catheter angiogram in 6 months to ensure that the sac remains occluded.

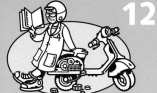

Children with a documented urinary tract infection (UTI) need to be investigated promptly and thoroughly, remembering the radiation dose that such examinations entail. The goals of imaging in UTI are to aid in the diagnosis of acute pyelonephritis, to identify those children who are at high risk of developing permanent renal damage and to confirm and monitor the presence of renal scarring. Conditions which are associated with the development of long-term renal damage include obstructive uropathies (e.g. pelvi-ureteric junction obstruction), renal calculi and congenital dysplastic kidneys.

UTIs are a common cause of morbidity in children. The term UTI, however, encompasses several different clinical conditions:

- Bacteriuria is defined as a colony count of $>10^5$/ml in a 'clean catch' (midstream, catheter or suprapubic aspirate) specimen of urine.
- A lower UTI is diagnosed clinically when there is dysuria, frequency of micturition and suprapubic tenderness in the absence of pyrexia.
- Acute pyelonephritis (APN) or an upper UTI is diagnosed when there is flank or abdominal pain, vomiting and a pyrexia $>38.5°C$, with cloudy or foul-smelling urine.
- The distinction between upper and lower urinary tract infections is clinically difficult but important, as permanent renal damage (scarring) may occur when the UTI involves the kidneys. There is an increased incidence of hypertension, complications during pregnancy and renal failure in adulthood in those who develop renal scars as a child.

The current imaging guidelines as recommended by the Royal College of Paediatrics and Child Health (RCPCH) are outlined in Figure 12.1. Local policies may vary somewhat.

Renal tract ultrasound

Ultrasound (US) defines the renal anatomy and will demonstrate any congenital abnormality such as a duplex or horseshoe kidney. Calculi are seen as

RCPCH imaging guidelines for urinary tract infection in childhood	
Age of patient	Imaging investigations required*
<2 years	Renal tract US, MCUG, DMSA
2–5 years	Renal tract US, DMSA†
>5 years	Renal tract US†

* Proven Proteus infection requires that an AXR be performed as Proteus sp. are associated with the formation of renal calculi.

† Micturating cystourethrography (MCUG) is also performed if the renal tract ultrasound (US) shows a hydroureter or if the dimercaptosuccinic acid (DMSA) scan is abnormal.

Fig. 12.1 RCPCH imaging guidelines for urinary tract infection in childhood.

echogenic (bright/white) foci. Scars may be seen as focal thinning of the renal cortex (more common in the upper and lower poles) or as a global reduction in the size of the kidney. Hydronephrosis is present when the renal pelvis and calyces are dilated, and the transverse diameter of the renal pelvis exceeds 1.0 cm. Neuropathic bladders are irregular in contour with thickened walls. Any sacculations and diverticula are seen as out-pouchings from the bladder wall.

Micturating cystourethrogram (MCUG)

A urinary catheter is inserted into the bladder and water-soluble contrast medium is then used to fill the bladder. Intermittent fluoroscopic images are obtained during bladder filling and micturition and demonstrate the outline of the bladder and the urethral contour (especially important in male infants). Vesico-ureteric reflux (VUR) is present when contrast flows retrogradely up the ureter(s) as the bladder is filled or during micturition (see Fig. 25.11). VUR is graded I–V depending on its severity.

DMSA

Tc^{99m} dimercaptosuccinic acid (DMSA) is administered intravenously. The dose depends on the child's weight. After 2 hours, images are obtained. The renal anatomy is demonstrated, as any functioning renal tissue will be outlined on the DMSA images. Renal scars manifest as defects in the renal outlines. The relative function of each kidney can be expressed as a percentage figure.

Other renal imaging investigations used in children with UTIs

VUR may also be detected directly by a nuclear cystogram, where pertechnetate is instilled directly into the bladder via a urinary catheter or indirectly when the child is imaged during micturition following an intravenous injection of Tc-labelled MAG-3.

CT scans may be helpful when renal infection is thought to have spread beyond the capsule of the kidney or when the child has been infected with an unusual organism, such as Candida sp. or *Mycobacterium tuberculosis*. MRI is increasingly used in the detection of renal scarring.

The role of vesico-ureteric reflux

VUR occurs due to an inadequate length of the intravesical ureter. The natural history is for spontaneous cessation of VUR in the majority of children, vesico-ureteric junction competence developing with an increase in the length of the submucosal ureteric tunnel.

The relationship between APN and VUR is not clear cut. VUR is reported to occur in 1–2% of healthy children and in almost two-thirds of children with UTIs. Importantly, there is an increased incidence of VUR in parents and siblings of children with reflux. VUR is also found in children with congenital and anatomical renal tract abnormalities. Such conditions include multicystic dysplastic kidney, pelvi-ureteric junction obstruction and duplex renal systems. Finally, VUR is also found in children who have bladder outlet obstruction, and neuropathic or dysfunctional bladders.

Studies have shown that more severe VUR, in association with APN, is more likely to result in the development of renal scars. However, not all children with VUR will develop renal damage, and some children with APN who go on to develop renal scars do not have demonstrable VUR. To further complicate the issue, some children with VUR will develop renal scarring in the absence of UTI.

In other words, when there is VUR, both sterile and infected urine may be associated with the development of renal scars, but VUR is not a prerequisite for the development of renal damage in children with a history of APN.

Case conference

A 4-month-old neonate was admitted last night with a 5-day history of vomiting and irritability. On examination he was dehydrated and his temperature was 39.5°C. He was tender to palpation in the left flank. His white cell count, ESR and CRP were all elevated. His urine was cloudy and malodorous. It contained numerous pus cells. He was resuscitated with IV fluids and commenced on empirical antibiotic therapy. A suprapubic bladder tap was performed and the clean urine sample sent to microbiology for culture.

Renal tract ultrasound
The images show dilatation of the pelvi-calyceal systems and ureters bilaterally. On the right side there is a single collecting system. On the left side there is a duplex collecting system, with complete duplication of the ureters to the level of the bladder. Both moieties of the duplex system are dilated. Posterior to the bladder all three dilated ureters can be seen. In addition, there is a soft tissue mass within the bladder, entered by one of the left-sided ureters. This is an ectopic ureterocoele associated with the upper moiety of a duplex system. The collecting systems and ureters are filled with echogenic debris. This likely represents pyoureteronephrosis.

In a young male infant such as this, you also need to consider whether there is a bladder outlet obstruction, such as that caused by posterior urethral valves. Other than the ureterocoele, the bladder appears normal on the ultrasound.

A micturating cystourethrogram (MCUG) should be performed to define the anatomy of the bladder and the urethra. The MCUG will also ascertain if the infant is refluxing into the dilated ureters.

Micturating cystourethrogram
The MCUG shows a filling defect on the left side of the bladder on the early filling views, consistent with the ureterocoele seen on the ultrasound images. The bladder outline is otherwise normal and, when the infant voided, the urethra was seen to be normal in contour. During bladder filling, however, there was VUR into both the right renal tract and the lower moiety of the left renal tract at low volumes. The ureters are dilated bilaterally and the calyces are clubbed. This corresponds to grade IV VUR. There was no VUR into the upper moiety system of the left kidney, confirming that it is obstructed by the ureterocoele.

- *Paediatric urologist*: I was asked to review this patient following his MCUG. His temperature has now settled on the antibiotic therapy. The urine cultures grew *Escherichia coli*. The patient is having a cystoscopy this afternoon, where we plan to incise the ureterocoele to release the obstruction.
- *Paediatric radiologist*: This infant has had bilateral pyoureteronephrosis associated with a left-sided duplex system. He has bilateral dilating VUR. He is at increased risk for the development of renal scarring. I would suggest a DMSA scan in 6 months' time to look for this. If he has further urinary tract infections, then the first-line investigation will be a repeat ultrasound examination.

13. Delayed Passage of Meconium

The vast majority of infants will pass meconium within the first 24 hours of life, and all should have done so by 48 hours of age. Delayed passage of meconium is normally associated with abdominal distension and vomiting (which may be bilious). In these circumstances, a supine abdominal radiograph and a contrast enema are indicated. The enema may be both diagnostic and therapeutic.

Figure 13.1 lists some of the more common causes of delayed passage of meconium in a newborn infant.

 Think anatomically from the anal verge extending proximally. This will help you to remember both the anatomical and functional abnormalities which cause a neonatal low bowel obstruction.

Hirschsprung's disease

Hirschsprung's disease is a form of functional low bowel obstruction which is due to failure of caudal migration of neuroblasts in the developing bowel. The distal large bowel from the point of neuronal arrest to the anus is aganglionic. In about 75% of cases, the aganglionic segment extends only to the rectosigmoid region (short segment disease). Long segment disease involves a variable portion of the colon proximal to the sigmoid, and total aganglionosis coli the entire colon and a part of the terminal ileum. Approximately 5% of children with Hirschsprung's disease have Down's syndrome (see Fig. 25.5).

Severe bloody diarrhoea, sepsis and shock are associated with Hirschsprung's enterocolitis, which occurs in up to 30% of patients in both the pre- and postoperative period. Enterocolitis is the leading cause of death in Hirschsprung's disease and has an increased frequency in long segment disease. A suction or full thickness rectal biopsy is required for the definitive diagnosis of Hirschsprung's disease.

Meconium ileus

Meconium ileus is a form of distal intestinal obstruction caused by inspissated pellets of meconium in the terminal ileum. Over 90% of infants with meconium ileus have cystic fibrosis, and meconium ileus is the presenting feature of cystic fibrosis in 10–15% of affected patients. Of all patients with cystic fibrosis, those with the $\Delta F508$ mutation (the commonest) have a higher incidence of meconium ileus.

Over half of the affected infants have uncomplicated meconium ileus. In utero these babies produce meconium that is thick and tenacious, and which fills and distends the small bowel loops. The meconium desiccates in the terminal ileum and becomes impacted, causing a high grade obstruction. A functional microcolon results. Meconium ileus is described as complicated when intra-uterine volvulus, atresia, gangrene, perforation or meconium peritonitis supervenes.

Functional immaturity of the colon

Immature left colon (also known as meconium plug syndrome or small left colon) is a relatively common cause of neonatal bowel obstruction.

Risk factors include premature infants, those born by caesarean section, maternal diabetes and drug ingestion, and infants whose mothers were treated with magnesium sulphate (for pre-eclampsia) during labour. The condition is *not* associated with cystic fibrosis. The exact cause of the syndrome remains unknown, but immaturity of the myenteric plexus had been postulated as a theory.

Delayed passage of meconium
• Hirschsprung's disease
• Meconium ileus
• Functional immaturity of the colon
• Ileal or colonic atresia
• Anorectal malformations
• Small bowel malrotation and volvulus
• Omphalomesenteric duct remnants
• Extrinsic compression of the distal bowel by a mass lesion
• Paralytic ileus, sepsis, drugs and metabolic upset

Fig. 13.1 Delayed passage of meconium.

	VACTERL*
V	Vertebral segmentation anomalies
A	Anorectal malformation
C	Congenital heart disease
T	Tracheo-oesophageal fistula
E	oEsophageal atresia
R	Renal anomalies
L	Limb anomalies (typically radial ray defects)

* Two or more components of the VACTERL sequence of malformations must be present for the infant to be labelled as belonging to this group.

Fig. 13.2 VACTERL.

Ileal atresia

Jejunal and ileal atresias have a common aetiology and are due to an intrauterine vascular accident. As with the duodenum, atresia is more common than stenosis, and the proximal jejunum and distal ileum are more frequently affected.

Anorectal malformations

The incidence of anorectal malformations (also known as imperforate anus or anorectal atresia) varies between 1 in 1500 and 1 in 5000 live births. The precise aetiology is unknown, but the condition results from failure of descent and separation of the hindgut and the genito-urinary tract during the second trimester. The abnormality consists of anorectal atresia, with or without an anomalous connection between the atretic anorectum and the genito-urinary tract.

Associated congenital anomalies are common. The VACTERL sequence occurs in around 45% of patients (Fig. 13.2).

Anorectal atresias are classified into high or low lesions depending upon whether the rectum ends above or below the puborectalis sling. The distinction between high and low lesions is clinical rather than radiological, and has important therapeutic and prognostic consequences.

In both males and females with low lesions, there is usually a visible perineal opening. The orifice may be located more anteriorly than normal (an ectopic anus) and it may be stenotic or covered with a membrane. Low lesions do not have a communication with the genito-urinary tract. Females with low lesions will have separate urethral and vaginal orifices with an intact hymen. Low lesions also include isolated rectal atresia or stenosis. This type of lesion is treated surgically with an anoplasty or dilatation soon after birth.

In both males and females with high lesions, no visible perineal fistula is present. Male patients will usually have a fistulous tract between the atretic anorectum and the posterior urethra. Less commonly there is a fistula to the bladder or anterior urethra. Female patients have fistulae from the atretic anorectum to the vagina or vestibule. Rarely, in both male and female patients, the rectum ends blindly. High lesions are initially managed with a colostomy to divert the faecal stream away from the genito-urinary tract. Definitive repair is performed at a later stage.

Colonic atresia

Colon atresia is rare when compared with other intestinal atresias, and colonic stenosis is rarer still. The right colon is most commonly affected.

It is thought to be due to an in utero vascular accident.

Radiological investigations

Abdominal x-ray (AXR)

This will show multiple, dilated loops of bowel down to the level of the obstruction, without distal gas. This appearance is referred to as a neonatal 'low bowel obstruction', i.e. the obstruction lies distal to the mid-ileum. In addition, there may or may not be a mottled faecal pattern seen in the right iliac fossa (the 'soap bubble' pattern; classically said to be diagnostic of meconium ileus, but is also seen with other causes of distal ileal obstruction).

Differentiation between small and large bowel on the AXR to determine the precise level of the obstruction is virtually impossible in the neonate. Both small and large bowel may be of similar calibre proximal to an obstruction, and the haustra are poorly developed in the neonatal bowel.

A neonatal 'high bowel obstruction' is present when the obstruction lies proximal to the mid-ileum. The AXR will show only a few dilated loops of bowel. Regardless of the cause, all neonates with a high bowel obstruction need urgent surgical referral, rather than further radiological investigation.

Contrast enema

It is important to ensure that the infant is fully resuscitated prior to the examination, and that IV fluids continue to run during the procedure. Water-soluble contrast medium is used, all types of which are hypertonic to the infant's plasma, placing the baby at risk of dehydration due to osmolar fluid shifts.

A supine view of the abdomen is initially required to exclude a complicating perforation. With the infant in the left lateral position, the tip of a Foley catheter is inserted just inside the anal margin. A small amount of contrast is hand injected. At this stage of the examination the radiologist is looking to exclude rectosigmoid Hirschsprung's disease. The following signs are present on the enema in this condition:

- There is a funnel-shaped zone of transition between the more proximal dilated (ganglionated) bowel and the distal narrow (denervated) bowel.
- The rectosigmoid ratio is reversed (i.e. the sigmoid colon has a greater diameter than the rectum; normally, the rectum is the most distensible part of the bowel).
- Abnormal muscle contractions may be observed in the denervated distal bowel.

The catheter balloon must never be inflated early on during the enema. At best the transition zone in Hirschsprung's disease would be missed and, at worst, a stiff, aganglionic rectum would be perforated.

If a low, rectosigmoid Hirschsprung's disease is excluded, the catheter may be inserted further and its balloon gently inflated, to act as a seal and prevent contrast leakage. The baby is placed supine and further contrast is injected. In all other causes of a low obstruction, the colon distal to the point of obstruction will be reduced in calibre. This is known as a *microcolon* and is due to colonic disuse in utero. The aim of the enema is to discover the precise level of the obstruction and, if possible, to run the contrast into the dilated, meconium-laden loops of bowel proximal to the point of obstruction. The enema then becomes both therapeutic and diagnostic. Water is drawn into the bowel lumen by osmosis, mixes with the tenacious meconium, loosens it and allows it to pass.

Infants with meconium ileus and functional immaturity of the colon will generally pass large quantities of meconium immediately following a successful enema, and their obstruction is relieved. Failure to relieve the bowel obstruction in meconium ileus may necessitate a second enema in the following days. Should this also fail to relieve the infant's symptoms, then surgery would usually be required. All infants with bowel atresias, stenoses, webs and Hirschsprung's disease need surgical intervention.

In an infant with functional immaturity of the colon, there is generally an abrupt change in colonic calibre seen at the level of the splenic flexure. It can be difficult to distinguish this condition from long segment Hirschsprung's disease with a transition zone at this level, and biopsy may later be required to confirm the presence of ganglion cells in the descending colon.

Case conference

The surgical team were asked to review a 2-day-old term neonate in the nursery by the paediatricians. The history was of progressive abdominal distension, failure to pass meconium and onset of bilious vomiting.

Abdominal radiographs
The supine abdominal x-ray demonstrates several distended loops of bowel throughout the abdomen. There is no gas seen in the rectum. It is impossible in a neonate to tell whether the distended loops are small or large bowel, as the valvulae conniventes and haustral pattern have not yet developed. However, given the number of dilated loops, the picture is that of a low bowel obstruction, i.e. the obstruction lies between the distal ileum and the anorectum. Low bowel obstructions in neonates should be investigated with a contrast enema. The enema is useful to determine the cause of the obstruction, be it mechanical or functional. In certain circumstances it may also be therapeutic.

(Neonatal contrast enemas are performed using a water-soluble contrast medium that is hypertonic to the infant's plasma. In cases of mechanical obstruction due to inspissated meconium, such as meconium ileus, the hypertonic fluid will draw extracellular water into the bowel lumen by osmosis and loosen off the meconium plugging the bowel lumen. In successful enemas, the infant will then pass this meconium and the obstruction will be relieved.)

Contrast enema
The enema images show an extremely narrow calibre colon. This is a microcolon—the colon of disuse. Contrast was run proximally to the caecum and refluxed through the ileocaecal valve into the terminal ileum. The ileum outlined by the contrast is also reduced in calibre. Only a few centimetres of small bowel are delineated and the contrast did not reach the dilated bowel loops. The implication is that the obstruction is mechanical and in the distal ileum. In meconium ileus we would expect to see filling defects in the bowel lumen of the terminal ileum due to the meconium pellets and to be able to run the contrast into the dilated bowel loops proximal to the luminal obstruction. This is not true of this case and therefore the radiological diagnosis is one of distal ileal atresia.

- *Paediatric surgeon*: This is generally an isolated congenital abnormality due to an ischaemic bowel injury. This may be a primary vascular accident or possibly secondary to an in utero mechanical obstruction such as a volvulus. The baby is scheduled for a laparotomy this afternoon.

14. A Limp in Childhood

Children not infrequently present with an inability to weight bear or a limp. The limp may be secondary to pain, or a structural hip or lower limb deformity. Clinically, it is important to try to localize any pain the child may have. Associated symptoms (such as fever) should be recorded and the time course of the symptoms noted. Radiologically, the commonest causes of a limp tend to be classified according to anatomic regions and the age of the patient. Some of the more common causes of a limp are outlined in Figure 14.1 and discussed in brief.

Developmental dysplasia of the hip (DDH)

The term developmental dysplasia of the hip (DDH) refers to an abnormal relationship between the femoral head and the acetabulum. Most cases of DDH are thought to be due to ligamentous laxity and a high level of maternal oestrogens. Risk factors include a positive family history, an abnormal position in utero, being of Caucasian racial origin or being papoosed with the hips in adduction, such as is traditional with Native American infants. Girls are much more commonly affected than boys. DDH is bilateral in up to one-third of cases. DDH may be clinically suspected if there are asymmetric gluteal folds, foot deformities or a positive Ortolani or Barlow test. Infants are usually screened if there is a positive family history or if they have been born by breech delivery.

Ultrasound of the hips is the imaging method of choice in young infants (see Fig. 25.6). In those children who have ossified femoral heads, an anteroposterior (AP) radiograph of the pelvis is performed. This is the first investigation used in those children who present late. The acetabular roof is steep and the femoral head is displaced superolaterally in infants with dysplastic hip joints. In addition, the ossification centre for the femoral head is small on the affected side.

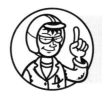 Non-ionising radiation techniques should be maximized in children.

Transient synovitis of the hip joint

Transient synovitis (irritable hip) is a common, non-traumatic cause of a limp in the younger child. The cause is unknown and the onset of symptoms acute. A hip joint effusion is present in the majority of patients. The diagnosis is one of

Common causes of a limp	
Age of patient	**Causes of a limp**
Up to 3 years	Developmental dysplasia of the hip, transient synovitis, septic arthritis, discitis, neuromuscular disorders
3–10 years	Perthes' disease, discitis (especially preschool children), inflammatory arthritides, Blount's disease
Adolescents	Slipped capital femoral epiphysis, discitis
Any age	Trauma, osteomyelitis, leg length discrepancy, bone tumours

Fig. 14.1 Common causes of a limp.

exclusion, the differential diagnoses including septic arthritis, inflammatory arthritides, leukaemia and trauma. Ultrasound of the hip joints and plain radiographs are the initial imaging investigations. The latter will be normal in this group of patients. The joint fluid, if aspirated, is sterile in patients with transient synovitis. Management is by bed rest, together with analgesics if required.

Septic arthritis

Septic arthritis refers to a joint infection and is usually due to pyogenic organisms. In infants and young children, infection spreads from the metaphysis, via the epiphyseal plate, to the epiphysis and joint space. In older children, spread is from an adjacent focus of osteomyelitis.

Ultrasound and plain radiographs of the hips are taken initially. Ultrasound can also be used to guide aspiration of fluid from the joint, which can then be sent for microbacterial analysis. The plain films may be normal early in the course of the illness. Destruction of the epiphysis and dislocation of the hip may be seen later on and in complicated cases. Skeletal scintigraphy is useful to exclude an associated osteomyelitis, and would show increased uptake on all phases of a three-phase examination.

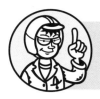

Septic arthritis requires urgent treatment to prevent joint destruction.

Perthes' disease

Perthes' disease (Legg–Calvé–Perthes' disease) is idiopathic avascular necrosis of the immature capital femoral epiphysis. The condition most commonly presents between the ages of 4 and 10 years, with boys being more often affected. Clinically, the child presents with hip or knee pain and a limp. The condition is bilateral in approximately 10% of cases.

Early changes in the bone include subchondral fissure fractures, and sclerosis and irregularity of the epiphysis. Later, the femoral head fragments

and collapses. The femoral neck may broaden and develop cystic change. Repair and re-ossification occur gradually, along with remodelling. The final contour of the bony epiphysis depends upon the original extent of the avascular necrosis and the patient's management. Initially, the patient is imaged using plain radiographs of the hips (see Fig. 25.14). MRI and isotope bone scans are helpful in the early stages if the plain films are normal. Bone marrow oedema can be demonstrated with MRI, and lack of femoral head enhancement following IV gadolinium (contrast) supports the diagnosis of avascular necrosis. At scintigraphy, lack of tracer uptake by the femoral head is seen with avascular necrosis. Treatment is aimed at keeping the femoral head contained by the acetabulum, protecting the articular cartilage and reducing the stress on the femoral head as it re-ossifies. Degenerative disease of the hip joint is a common late sequela.

Perthes' disease more commonly presents between the ages of 4 and 8 years; Slipped Capital Femoral Epiphysis (SCFE) occurs in adolescents.

Slipped capital femoral epiphysis (SCFE)

Slipped capital (or upper) femoral epiphysis (SCFE) is a hip disorder of adolescence. Most cases are regarded as idiopathic, although it is thought that it may be a hormone-mediated process, given its occurrence around the time of the pubertal growth spurt. In up to one-third of patients, SCFE is a bilateral, though asymmetric, condition.

The lesion of SCFE is analogous to a Salter I fracture across the proximal femoral growth plate. The femoral head slips posteriorly and medially. The abnormal position of the femoral head is best seen on the frog-leg lateral radiograph. The AP radiograph may be normal, or there may be subtle broadening of the growth plate and a reduced height of the femoral head (see Fig. 25.15). Further slippage is prevented by pinning of the femoral head in place (it is *not* manipulated back to the anatomical position). Chondrolysis of the articular cartilage of the femoral head and avascular necrosis are the two most significant complications and may occur pre- and post-pinning.

Toddler's fracture

Toddler's fracture is the synonym used to describe an undisplaced spiral or oblique tibial fracture that occurs in children between the ages of 9 months to 3 years when they are beginning to weightbear. These children present with a history of a limp or refusal to bear weight. A history of trauma may not be elicited. The initial radiographs are often normal. The children are usually treated symptomatically in a cast. Repeat x-rays after 10–14 days will confirm a healing fracture.

Discitis

Infection involving the intervertebral disc and/or the adjacent vertebral body endplates leads to severe back pain and muscle spasm. Limping is more common in younger children. The infection is usually low grade, with Staphylococcus as the underlying organism. Systemic signs tend to be minimal. Diagnosis is often difficult, as plain radiographs may be normal for several weeks. MRI is the most helpful imaging technique as it will confirm disc space narrowing and oedema of the adjacent vertebral bodies. Intravenous gadolinium is helpful in detecting complications such as a paravertebral or extradural abscess. Patients with discitis are treated with antibiotics, analgesics and bed rest.

Radiological evaluation

Pelvic radiographs
Two views of the hip joints are usually performed in children and adolescents. These are the straight AP view and the 'frog leg' lateral (Lowenstein) view. The knees are bent up and the hips are then abducted. Plain radiographs of the hips are taken in all children who present with a limp, unless there is a definite predisposing factor (e.g. trauma) or focal signs directing the clinician elsewhere, on clinical examination.

Radiographs of the lumbar spine
Lower back pain is a relatively common complaint in children and adolescents, usually due to soft tissue injury. Persistent back pain in this age group, however, is a symptom that must be taken seriously. Plain radiographs of the lumbar spine are the first-line imaging investigation, but it should be remembered that they are a high radiation dose examination. Radiographs are useful in the setting of trauma and also when looking for signs of inflammation (osteomyelitis and discitis), benign and malignant spinal tumours, and congenital spinal abnormalities (including scoliosis).

In the setting of persistent lower back pain with normal radiographs, the child should proceed to an isotope bone scan and/or an MRI of the lumbar spine.

Ultrasound scan of the hips
The best way of detecting a hip joint effusion is by ultrasound. Each hip is scanned in turn using a high frequency linear probe. The joint capsule is seen as an echogenic line, which normally runs parallel to the femoral neck. When a joint effusion is present, the joint capsule has a convex anterior margin, and the joint space is widened by the anechoic fluid. The depth of the effusion may be measured between the femoral neck and the joint capsule. A value greater than 4 mm or a difference between the two sides of greater than 2 mm is considered significant.

Ultrasound of the hips to look for dysplasia
This examination can only be performed in young infants before the femoral head has ossified (usually around 4–6 months of age). Each hip is scanned in turn using a high frequency linear probe. The ultrasound probe is held longitudinally over the hip joint. The iliac bone is seen in profile, along with the acetabular roof, triradiate cartilage, cartilaginous labrum and the unossified femoral head. The femoral head should be one-half to two-thirds covered by the acetabular roof, and the iliac bone and acetabulum should form a sharp angle together.

Isotope bone scans (scintigraphy)

Methylene diphosphonate (MDP) is labelled with Tc^{99m} and injected into the patient (see Part II, Principles of Radiology). The dose of the radiopharmaceutical administered is dependent upon the child's weight. The isotope is taken up in areas of active bone metabolism. The examination may be performed as either a three-phase or a static scan. In the former, images are obtained in the vascular (immediate), blood pool (after about 5 minutes) and static (after about 2 hours) phases. This type of scan is useful to investigate suspected inflammatory bone disease, infection or trauma.

A static scan alone is useful in the detection of both benign and malignant bone tumours, and also has a place in the investigation of children with lower back pain, osteomyelitis and Perthes' disease. When there is avascular necrosis, no isotope is taken up (a 'cold spot'). Magnification of the relevant areas with a pinhole collimator is a useful technique in paediatric patients, particularly in the assessment of lesions adjacent to the metabolically active epiphyseal plate. Tomographic scintigraphy (SPECT) is particularly helpful in the evaluation of spinal abnormalities.

CT scan of the hips

This is rarely done outside the setting of trauma. However, it is increasingly used in infants and older children with DDH who have had failed conservative management.

Infants with DDH occasionally have CT scans performed to confirm the correct position of the femoral heads relative to the acetabula, once they are in spica casts (plaster casts that hold the hips in abduction).

MRI of the hips and pelvis

Use of MRI tends to be reserved for those children in whom a diagnosis cannot be made by a combination of ultrasound, plain radiographs and scintigraphy, or those children with complications of their primary pathology. MRI has the advantage of not using ionising radiation, but has the disadvantage of requiring sedation or anaesthesia in younger children. It is particularly useful in examining the cartilaginous structures of the hip, such as the labrum in DDH. It is also useful, acutely, in children with suspected bone and joint infection or avascular necrosis of the femoral head.

 Isotope bone scans should always be interpreted alongside plain radiographs of the area under investigation.

Case conference

A 9-year-old boy originally presented with a 3-day history of severe left-sided hip pain and a limp. On examination, the left leg was held adducted and externally rotated. Passive abduction, flexion and internal rotation were all decreased. The child's past history revealed that he had complained of an ache in his left groin over the past 2 months. He was on regular peritoneal dialysis, having been born with posterior urethral valves and subsequently developing renal failure.

AP and Lowenstein views of both hips were obtained. These show an abnormal bone texture, with mixed areas of sclerosis and reduced bone density. There is widening of the proximal femoral growth plate on the right side and irregularity of the symphysis pubis. These features are consistent with renal osteodystrophy. On the left side, the femoral head has slipped posteriorly and medially. This is seen best on the Lowenstein view. The diagnosis is left-sided slipped capital (upper) femoral epiphysis, secondary to renal osteodystrophy.

The patient was taken to theatre and the epiphysis was pinned in place. That was 2 months ago. The patient has now re-presented with increasing pain in both hips.

- *Paediatric radiologist*: The new AP and Lowenstein views of the pelvis again show the bone changes of renal osteodystrophy. Two screws are seen along the left femoral neck, passing into the left femoral head. Note that the position of the left femoral head has not changed since the initial films, the pins having prevented further slippage of the epiphysis. However, the procedure has been complicated by the development of avascular necrosis (AVN) in the left capital femoral epiphysis. The height of the epiphysis is reduced, its outline is irregular and it is very sclerotic. On the right side, the capital femoral epiphysis has also started to slip; it has moved posteriorly and medially.
- *Orthopaedic surgeon*: The new slip of the right capital femoral epiphysis requires pinning. In addition, given the development of AVN in the left femoral head, the pins on the left side need to be removed or retracted to prevent the development of chondrolysis (articular cartilage necrosis of the femoral head).
- *Paediatric radiologist*: Given that he has renal osteodystrophy, he is at risk of epiphyseal slippage at other sites, particularly at the wrist. This should be borne in mind if he complains of pain in other joints.

15. Pregnancy

Obstetric ultrasound is used both for routine assessment to confirm pregnancy has occurred and that its milestones have been achieved. In addition, fetal and maternal abnormalities are assiduously checked for.

First trimester ultrasound

This is intended to fulfil the following functions:
- Confirmation of pregnancy.
- Confirmation of dates.
- Threatened abortion.
- Suspected multiple gestation.
- Suspected ectopic pregnancy.
- Screening for fetal abnormality.
- Molar pregnancy.

Confirmation of pregnancy

Ultrasound is used to determine the presence of the gestation sac, yolk sac, fetal pole (embryo), amnion and cardiac activity. The gestational sac is not visible until it is 2–3 mm in size (at 4.5 weeks) and it increases by 1 mm per day.

Transvaginal ultrasound scanning (TVUS) will demonstrate structures and confirm viability about 1 week earlier than transabdominal scanning (TAS).

TAS is performed initially but if its findings are inconclusive or too early to confirm viability, then TVUS is used. A full maternal bladder is essential for TAS in early pregnancy but must be empty for TVUS. The fetal pole should be reliably seen by weeks 5–6 on TVUS and by week 7 on TAS. Fetal cardiac activity should now be visible and a viable pregnancy can be confidently diagnosed.

Confirmation of dates

Clinical dating of a pregnancy is based on the patient's recollection of the first day of her last menstrual period (LMP) and on the estimation of uterine size. Both these methods are prone to inaccuracy.

Ultrasound milestones in the first trimester are a much more accurate means of assessing gestational age from 5 weeks onwards. The earliest accurate method is by measuring the gestational sac diameter, circumference or volume at 5–6 weeks.

After 6 weeks the fetal pole is reliably visualized and a crown–rump length (CRL) measurement is performed. CRL is the maximum length of the fetal pole from the top of the head to rump excluding limb buds and yolk sac. CRL measurement is accurate from 6–12 weeks (±5 days).

Threatened abortion

Threatened abortion is the association of vaginal bleeding and cramping within the first 20 weeks of pregnancy. The possible findings on ultrasound include:
- *Viable pregnancy*: A gestation sac with a viable fetal pole correctly implanted in the uterine cavity.
- *Incomplete abortion*: Some of the products of conception may have passed but the uterus may contain an ill-defined sac or mass. No viable fetus
- *Complete abortion*: An enlarged uterus in keeping with early pregnancy but no evidence of sac or fetal pole. Thickened decidual reaction may be visible in the endometrium.
- *Missed abortion*: The gestation sac and fetal pole are visible but there is no evidence of viability (a fetal pole larger than 5 mm should show cardiac activity).
- *Anembryonic pregnancy*: Blighted ovum, in which the sac develops but the fetus does not. Ultrasound demonstrates an empty sac, usually larger than expected for dates. A mean sac diameter greater than 2.5 cm and no fetal pole

is diagnostic of a blighted ovum (TAS). A small empty sac could be due to incorrect dates. If the diagnosis is in doubt, either use TVUS or rescan TAS in 7–10 days.

Suspected multiple gestation

Check for the presence of more than one gestational sac (dizygotic/fraternal) or more than one fetal pole in a single sac (monozygotic/identical). Multiple pregnancies have an incidence of 1%, of which approximately two-thirds are dizygotic/polyzygotic.

In early first trimester, bleeding at the site of implantation may mimic a second sac—two fetal poles should be identified before making the diagnosis of multiple pregnancy. It is important to determine chorionicity in early pregnancy due to the higher incidence of fetal abnormalities and complications in monochorionic pregnancy.

Between 6 and 9 weeks, dichorionic twins have a thick separating membrane >2 mm in diameter. After 9 weeks the membrane becomes progressively thinner and measurement less reliable. In dichorionic twins the junction of the membrane with the sac wall gives a characteristic 'lambda' sign.

When one sac is identified, search for two. When two sacs are identified, search for three, and so on . . .

Suspected ectopic pregnancy

The patient will present with a positive pregnancy test, pelvic pain, abnormal vaginal bleeding and will possibly be in shock. There may be a clinical suspicion of a pelvic mass. If ultrasound shows an intrauterine pregnancy, then a coexistent ectopic is highly unlikely (incidence of 1 in 30,000). Possible US findings are of a complex adnexal mass with fluid in the pouch of Douglas (blood) and a fluid collection in the endometrium (pseudosac).

TVUS may show an extrauterine sac with a live embryo. This is conclusive of an ectopic pregnancy but only represents 5% of cases.

Screening for fetal abnormality

Ultrasound can be used to measure the nuchal translucency (NT) at the back of the fetal neck.

An NT >3 mm increases the fetal risk for chromosomal abnormalities, especially trisomy 21 (Down's syndrome). NT is usually used in conjunction with maternal age and biochemical triple screening to assess an individual's risk. Counselling on the risk value is an integral part of the test.

Ultrasound may also demonstrate some gross fetal abnormalities, such as anencephaly, towards the end of the first trimester.

Molar pregnancy (gestational trophoblastic disease)

The patient may present with painless vaginal bleeding, excessive vomiting and high blood pressure.

US will show a uterus filled with an endometrial mass with or without cystic spaces ('snowstorm' appearance). In 50% of cases large cysts containing septa may be present in the ovaries (theca luteal cysts). These are thought to be due to increased levels of circulating human chorionic gonadotrophin (HCG). Occasionally an anembryonic sac may be seen.

Molar pregnancy can be partial or complete. Partial moles may have a coexistent fetus or fetal parts but these are not present in a complete molar pregnancy. Although benign, molar pregnancies may predispose to an invasive mole or the development of choriocarcinoma.

Second trimester ultrasound

Indications include:
- Assess fetal normality.
- Confirmation of dates.
- Adjunct to amniocentesis.
- Raised maternal serum alphafetoprotein.

Assess fetal normality

US is an essential tool in detecting major and minor fetal structural abnormalities and requires a skilled and experienced operator. It will not detect all fetal abnormalities. It must be performed before 24 weeks if termination of pregnancy is an option. It is commonly offered to all pregnant mothers as part of a screening test in association with maternal serum alphafetoprotein levels (MSAFP) levels. Anomalies detectable by US are as follows.

Neural tube defects (NTDs)
Incidence of 5 per 1000 births; predominantly anencephaly and spina bifida (SB) (95%).

Anencephaly
Absence of cranial vault and cerebral hemispheres. Evident on view for biparietal diameter (BPD) and sagittal section. Fetus still moves and kicks. May have associated spinal lesions (50%). Can be diagnosed after 11 weeks.

Encephalocele
Five percent of NTDs. Defect in cranium usually occipital (75%) with associated herniated fluid-filled or brain-filled cysts.

Spina bifida
Usually detected by recognizing associated defects in the skull, which act as markers: frontal bone scalloping ('lemon' sign) and/or anterior elongated curvature of the cerebellum ('banana' sign). Spina bifida is visible as widening of the fetal spine with a posterior cyst, filled with either fluid or spinal cord. Ventriculomegaly is usually present.

Cranial disorders
Ventriculomegaly
Increase in size of ventricles, usually lateral. Early enlargement is diagnosed by measuring the diameter at the level of the atrium (abnormal >10mm). Incidence of 2 per 1000 births. It is usually caused by obstruction which may be internal or external.

Dandy–Walker syndrome
Visible on US as a large posterior fossa cyst (dilated fourth ventricle). The cerebellum may be splayed with the vermis absent. Incidence of 1 per 30,000 births.

Agenesis of the corpus callosum (CC)
The CC is composed of nerve fibres connecting two cerebral hemispheres at the cavum septum pellucidum (CSP). Absence of CSP at BPD level may indicate diagnosis.

Holoprosencephaly
The brain fails to divide into two halves, resulting in little or no visible midline echo (falx). A single dilated lateral ventricle is visible. There are three main types depending on the degree of cleavage: lobar, semi-lobar and alobar.

Microcephaly
Small brain, small head. Diagnosed by serial measurements of head to abdomen circumference ratios.

Cardiac disorders
This is the largest group of congenital abnormalities and accounts for 1% of all abnormalities at birth. They range in severity and may be isolated or associated with other conditions. Diagnosis depends on the demonstration of the four chambers and right and left outflow tracts on a transverse section of the fetal heart. It is important to recognize the foramen ovale as a normal defect between the atria and that the normal fetal heart rate is 120–160 bpm.

The conditions outlined in Figure 15.1 are potentially detectable using US.

Thoracic disorders
Cystic adenomatoid malformation (CAM)
A condition of the fetal lung involving the development of cysts of various sizes. Usually unilateral (85%).

Lung sequestration
A bright mass usually located in the lower lobes of the lung may correspond to a sequestrated lobe. This lobe has a separate blood supply and has no connection to the airways.

Cardiac conditions potentially detectable using ultrasound
• Dextrocardia
• Atrial and ventricular septal defects
• Univentricular heart
• Hypoplastic left ventricle
• Pulmonary stenosis and atresia
• Transposition of the great vessels
• Tetralogy of Fallot
• Ebstein's anomaly
• Double outlet ventricle
• Dysrhythmias—ectopics, supraventricular tachycardia, complete heart block

Fig. 15.1 Cardiac conditions potentially detectable using ultrasound.

Pleural effusion

Appearance of fluid at the base of the fetal lungs—may be either unilateral or bilateral ('batwing' appearance). May be associated with other conditions such as hydrops fetalis.

Diaphragmatic hernia

Incidence of 1 per 4000 births. Although the diaphragm is difficult to image, the associated pathology will lead to the diagnosis. Check for the position of the fetal stomach: if a cystic mass is present in the thorax and no stomach is seen in the left upper abdomen then a left-sided hernia is present. The heart is also displaced to the right. Left-sided hernia is more common than right-sided.

Abdominal disorders

These may be divided into three main groups: abdominal wall, gastrointestinal tract and urinary tract.

Abdominal wall defects

Exomphalos   This is characterized by a sac anterior to the abdominal wall, covered by a layer of peritoneum. The sac contains solid and cystic components representing the liver, stomach and bowel. It is a midline defect and the umbilical cord enters at the apex of the sac. Check for other fetal abnormalities.

Gastroschisis   An isolated condition in which a defect is present, usually to the right of the cord insertion. Fetal bowel can be seen freely floating in the amniotic fluid. There is no covering membrane.

Gastrointestinal disorders

Abnormalities of the gastrointestinal system usually result in increased amniotic fluid levels (polyhydramnios) due to impaired fetal swallowing.

Oesophageal atresia   In 10% of cases complete atresia results in no stomach being visible on US, and associated polyhydramnios. The majority of cases have an associated tracheo-oesophageal fistula which may cause the stomach to fill and make antenatal diagnosis difficult.

Duodenal and jejunal atresia   A double or triple bubble appearance in the upper abdomen caused by a dilated proximal gastrointestinal tract.

Abdominal cysts   Fluid-filled cysts may be identified in the fetal abdomen arising from the liver, biliary tree (choledochal cysts), ovary or mesentery.

Urinary tract disorders

Obstructive lesions are associated with reduced amniotic fluid (oligohydramnios). Normal US must show both kidneys and a fluid-filled bladder. Abnormalities range from simple cysts to lethal conditions.

Renal agenesis   Bilateral agenesis is lethal. Failure to show the fetal bladder (no urine production) or either kidney with no amniotic fluid is consistent with the diagnosis. Incidence of 1 per 5000 births. May be unilateral (1 per 2000 births). Affected babies have a normal prognosis.

Infantile polycystic kidney disease   Always bilateral. Appear as large echobright kidneys due to microcystic appearance.

Obstructive uropathies   This describes a large range of conditions and US appearances. There may be mild unilateral renal dilatation to severe bilateral hydronephrosis caused by urethral stenosis. US will demonstrate fluid in the renal collecting systems with reduced levels of renal cortical tissue and decreased amniotic fluid.

Skeletal disorders

Ultrasound can demonstrate conditions that cause limb shortening or absence of all or part of a limb.

Confirmation of dates

Fetal biometry can be performed during the second trimester to confirm the menstrual dates and set a delivery date. Confirmation of dates is also essential for any follow-up growth scans. The routine measurements performed are as follows.

Biparietal diameter

Performed on a transverse section of the fetal skull at the level of the CSP, thalami, midline echo and complete symmetrical cranium (see Fig. 25.16). The ultrasound's calipers are positioned perpendicular to the midline from the outer aspect of the upper parietal bone to the inner aspect of the opposite side.

Head circumference (HC)

Measured on the same section as the BPD. A trace is performed around the outer aspect of the cranium.

Abdominal circumference (AC)

A transverse section measured at the level of the stomach and intrahepatic portion of the umbilical vein (see Fig. 25.17). It is used in the third trimester to assess growth and to estimate fetal weight.

Femur length (FL)

A full-length view of the femur is obtained and calipers placed at each end (see Fig. 25.18). BPD and FL should correspond.

Adjunct to amniocentesis

Ultrasound is used pre-, post- and often during amniocentesis and other invasive procedures. Pre-procedure it is used to assess fetal position, the location of the placenta and to locate an accessible pool of amniotic fluid. Needle insertion and guidance can be imaged in real time using ultrasound.

Raised maternal serum alphafetoprotein (MSAFP)

Alphafetoprotein is produced by the fetal liver and reaches a peak in amniotic fluid at 16–18 weeks and in maternal blood at 32 weeks. It may be used as part of a screening test for fetal abnormalities. A raised MSAFP should result in a detailed scan of fetal anatomy.

Causes of raised MSAFP include:
- Neural tube defects— anencephaly, spina bifida, encephalocoele.
- Abdominal wall defects.
- Gastrointestinal tract abnormalities.
- Other abnormalities, e.g. cleft palate.
- Wrong dates.
- Twins.
- Fetal demise.

Third trimester ultrasound

Indications include:
- Small for dates.
- Large for dates.
- Fetal distress.
- Vaginal bleeding.

Small for dates

The fetus may be small for dates because of incorrect dates and gestation being less than expected, difficulty in assessing gestation from palpation due to obesity of the mother, intrauterine growth retardation (IUGR) and reduced amniotic fluid (oligohydramnios).

IUGR

A fetus has IUGR when it is below the tenth centile for weight at any given gestational age or is less than 2.5 kg at 36 weeks. It is important to differentiate between a baby that is small for dates but normal, and one that is growth retarded. There are two main forms of IUGR:

- *Symmetrical*: The entire fetus is smaller than normal. Common causes include chromosomal abnormality, intrauterine viral infection, chronic maternal illness or drug intake (smoking, alcohol). The diagnosis requires accurate dating at an early stage (first trimester or 18–22 week scan) and third trimester serial measurements of fetal head and trunk. Common measurements are HC and AC. Symmetrical IUGR will show a progressive fall off in growth for both parameters over time when compared to normal tables.
- *Asymmetrical*: The fetal trunk is small but the head is normal in size (brain sparing). It is caused by placental insufficiency. HC/AC ratio is needed to confirm the diagnosis (rule out hydrocephalus as another cause of high HC/AC—a low ratio may indicate microcephaly).

Oligohydramnios

Oligohydramnios is defined as a liquor pool less than 2 cm in depth. Causes include renal anomalies such as renal agenesis (check for the presence of the fetal bladder—excludes renal agenesis), neural tube defects and premature rupture of the membranes (US is useful in not only showing reduced liquor but also the size of the fetus, and whether a fetal anomaly is present. An anomaly with an associated polyhydramnios may have caused the membranes to rupture).

Large for dates

The causes include polyhydramnios, multiple gestation, macrosomia, incorrect dates and uterine masses.

Polyhydramnios

Polyhydramnios is defined as a liquor pool greater than 8 cm.

Causes of polyhydramnios are outlined in Figure 15.2.

Multiple gestation

Problems associated with multiple pregnancies include IUGR, polyhydramnios, preterm delivery and placenta praevia. There is an increased incidence of fetal abnormality, particularly with monozygotic twins.

Macrosomia

Macrosomia is defined as a baby larger than 4 kg at birth, and this can cause problems during delivery. There is an association with maternal diabetes. The diagnosis is made with serial AC measurements. There may be associated polyhydramnios.

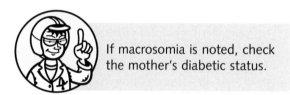

If macrosomia is noted, check the mother's diabetic status.

Incorrect dates

A mother presenting late in pregnancy may actually be at a later gestation than menstrual dates suggest.

Uterine masses

The presence of fibroids may cause uterine enlargement. US will demonstrate a solid mass within the uterine wall. Occasionally, fibroids may

change in appearance as a result of cystic degeneration or bleeding (red degeneration). Scan should also check for maternal ovarian masses, which are predominantly cystic.

Fetal hydrops

This is characterized on US by fetal ascites, skin and scalp oedema, pleural effusion, pericardial effusion and polyhydramnios. If the placenta is thickened, Rhesus incompatibility (immune hydrops) is the likely cause. Other causes (non-immune hydrops) include fetal cardiac and chest abnormalities, infections (toxoplasmosis, rubella) and chromosomal disease.

Fetal distress

The fetus may be at risk of distress or death due to conditions such as:
- Maternal—chronic hypertension, pre-eclampsia, diabetes mellitus and drug addiction.
- Fetal—presence of abnormality.
- Placental—insufficiency or fetal abruption.
- Previous history of stillbirth or distress.

Close monitoring of the fetus and its environment is essential to detect early signs of distress. Methods of detecting early distress include:
- *Biophysical profile*: A score is attributed to each of the following as observed over a 30-minute US scan: fetal breathing, fetal tone, fetal movement, amniotic fluid volume and fetal heart rate. Total possible score is 10. Some centres have also assessed the placenta for signs of early maturity.
- *Umbilical artery Doppler*: The umbilical artery is sampled using Doppler US to obtain a waveform trace. The diastolic portion of the waveform is related to vascular resistance in the placenta. Increased resistance will cause decreased, absent or reversed diastolic flow. Often the ratio of peak systolic to end diastolic is used to quantify this, i.e. the resistance index (RI). Abnormal findings on umbilical artery Doppler are associated with a poor outcome for the fetus.

Fetal death may occur in utero. US findings will vary depending on time since death (Fig. 15.3).

Vaginal bleeding

Placenta praevia is defined as a placenta that partially or totally covers the internal os and is

---

Causes of polyhydramnios

- Fetal abnormalities affecting the gastrointestinal tract and the CNS (if swallowing mechanism affected)
- Skeletal and abdominal wall defects
- Diabetic pregnancy
- Multiple gestation
- Fetal hydrops
- Infections (toxoplasmosis and rubella)

Fig. 15.2 Causes of polyhydramnios.

Ultrasound findings in fetal death

- No evidence of fetal cardiac activity
- Absent fetal movement
- Skin oedema
- Overlapping of skull bones (Spalding's sign)
- Biparietal diameter will decrease on subsequent scans
- Abnormal fetal position
- Fetal trunk appears collapsed

Fig. 15.3 Ultrasound findings in fetal death.

usually identified on the 18–22 week scan as a low-lying placenta. Most low-lying placentas identified on these early scans do not present as praevia because of subsequent placental 'migration'. Separation from the myometrium may cause vaginal bleeding. Transabdominal US (with an empty bladder) will show praevia. A full bladder may give the false impression of praevia by compressing the cervix and making it appear longer. Vaginal scanning can be used to demonstrate the lower uterine segment if TAS is undiagnostic.

Placental abruption is caused by all, or some, of the placenta separating from the myometrium before delivery. Major abruptions are diagnosed clinically; the role of US is to determine fetal viability. Minor abruptions appear as an echopoor mass (clot) between the placenta and the myometrium. Amniotic fluid may contain echoes representing blood. Bleeding may also occur in the subchorionic portion of the placenta (marginal bleed) or within the placental tissue (intraplacental bleed).

Case conference

A 28-year-old lady presents at 21 weeks' gestation with a raised maternal serum alphafetoprotein (MSAFP) as part of a routine biochemical analysis. Due to the increased incidence of fetal abnormality with raised MSAFP (in particular neural tube defects), a fetal anomaly scan was organized.

Ultrasound scan
Sagittal views of the fetus confirm viability with normal to increased fetal movement. Fetal trunk and limbs are identified but absence of the cranial vault is noted. Coronal views of the fetal face demonstrate a characteristic 'frogs' eyes' appearance. Transverse view for BPD again showed absence of bony skull (acrania) and cerebral hemispheres. The appearances are consistent with anencephaly.

The patient was referred for a tertiary level scan in the fetal medicine centre and for counselling. The provisional diagnosis of anencephaly is confirmed.

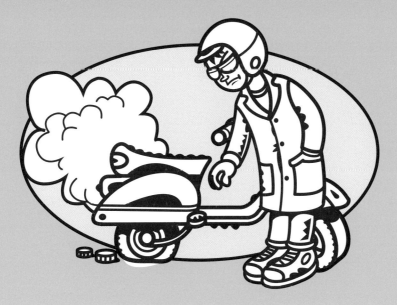

PRINCIPLES OF RADIOLOGY

16. Ionizing Radiation Studies

Radiology, or medical imaging, is a rapidly diversifying and increasingly pivotal discipline within medicine. Multiple imaging modalities are available. Some, e.g. CT, involve irradiation of the patient, and others, notably magnetic resonance and ultrasound, do not (Fig. 16.1).

Both the clinician and the radiologist involved in a patient's care should act to minimize any dose of ionizing radiation—the clinician, through requesting appropriate investigations based on clinical acumen, and the radiologist in choosing the most appropriate imaging modality to gain the necessary information to aid diagnosis and management.

This section considers the phenomena involved in the generation of radiological images. The terminology used to describe findings is dependent on the imaging method used (Fig. 16.1).

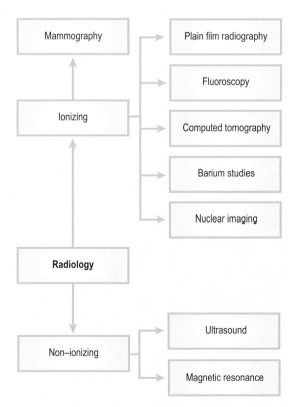

Fig. 16.1 Terminology of imaging modalities.

Conventional radiology

Production of x-rays

X-rays form part of the electromagnetic spectrum and are produced by heating a tungsten filament (the cathode) inside an evacuated tube (a vacuum). Electrons liberated from the cathode are focused on to an anode by creating a large potential difference between the two. X-ray photons are released from the anode by this electron bombardment. The casing of the x-ray tube absorbs most of the radiation, but a small proportion escapes through a window in the tube. This beam of radiation can be passed through the human body and detected by a photographic film (or digital imaging system). This film is sandwiched between two fluorescent screens. X-rays cause the emission of light from the screens and this light causes blackening of the film's emulsion once developed.

Radiographic appearances

It is possible to differentiate four separate tissues on radiographs because of their differential absorption of the x-ray beam (Fig. 16.2). All soft tissues, except fat, absorb the same amount of x-ray radiation and therefore appear the same shade of grey. Fat absorbs slightly less radiation than other soft tissues, and therefore looks a little darker. Bones absorb most radiation and therefore appear

Appearance on plain radiographs	
Colour	Tissue/artefact
Black	Gas
Dark grey	Fat
Grey	Soft tissues (except fat)
White	Bone
Intense white	Metallic objects

Fig. 16.2 Appearance on plain radiographs.

white, while air absorbs least and looks black. The fifth category is artefact, e.g. metallic foreign bodies, which appear as intense white foci on the radiograph.

Frontal chest radiograph (PA and AP projections)

The frontal chest radiograph is the most commonly requested radiological examination. The indications are diverse, but dyspnoea, chest pain and haemoptysis are common reasons for request.

Technically, the radiograph should be well centred with the medial borders of the clavicle equidistant from the spinous processes (see Fig. 19.1). A good inspiratory effort should be made, confirmed by identifying 10 ribs posteriorly at the level of the mid-clavicular line (see Fig. 19.2). It is mandatory to check the patient details and confirm that the name and the date of the examination are correct. Nipple markers can be useful (see Fig. 19.3).

When reviewing a chest film, a scheme of 'review areas' is indicated to ensure that all parts of the film are examined (Fig. 16.3).

Areas to review on the chest radiograph include:
• The cardiac silhouette
• The mediastinum
• The lung fields
• The costophrenic angles
• The diaphragm.

Lateral chest radiograph

The lateral chest radiograph may be useful for localizing, within the chest, a focal lesion (e.g. tumour) or artefact (e.g. pacing wires). One radiological maxim is that a pulmonary lesion not identified on the frontal chest radiograph is most unlikely to be seen on a lateral film. It should not be considered an alternative pulmonary imaging technique.

Apical chest radiograph

The apical radiograph is very useful in evaluating the upper aspects of each lung. This region is partially obscured by the clavicles and the upper ribs on the standard frontal chest radiograph. An apical view permits a clearer view of this region.

Abdominal radiograph

The supine abdominal film is commonly requested for the investigation of non-specific abdominal pain (Fig. 16.4).

Areas to review on the abdominal radiograph include:

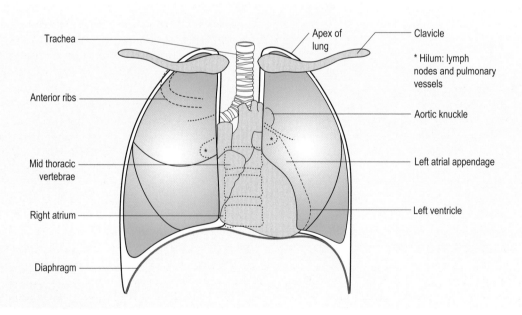

Fig. 16.3 Normal chest x-ray gross structures.

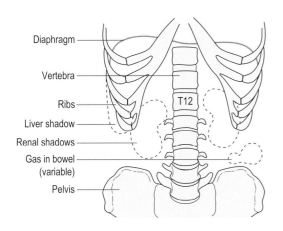

Fig. 16.4 Normal abdominal x-ray gross structures.

- Bowel gas pattern (intraluminal gas)
- Extraluminal gas
- Vertebral column and pelvis.

Features to look for

The bowel should be evaluated to exclude gaseous distension of the small and/or large bowel and evidence of extraluminal air, e.g. pneumoperitoneum, or bowel displacement by organomegaly. Renal or biliary calcification can also be demonstrated, as may bony pathology affecting the lower ribs, lumbar spinal column and the pelvis.

Spinal radiographs

Spinal radiographs are typically requested to exclude trauma or arthropathy of the vertebral bone and joint architecture. Typically frontal and lateral (orthogonal) views are performed.

Cervical spine

At the cervical level, dedicated 'peg views' are also used. Check for visibility of all seven cervical vertebrae and the upper border of the first thoracic vertebral body. Check the vertebral alignment and the disc spacing. Check the arcs (alignment of the anterior and posterior vertebral margins and the spinolaminar line), the width of the paravertebral soft tissues and the shape of the prepharyngeal space.

A C-spine *cannot* be cleared unless all seven cervical vertebrae and the first thoracic vertebra are seen.

Thoracic and lumbar spine

The main indications for these radiographs are back pain and following trauma. It is important to perform orthogonal (anterior and lateral) views. Check the vertebral alignment and the disc spacing, and the presence of pedicles (on the anterior view). Examine the apophyseal and the facet joints.

Limb x-rays

These are usually indicated to evaluate bone or joint pathology. Again orthogonal views are indicated. For symptomatology related to a bone, the joint at either end of that bone should be included on the radiograph.

Orthopaedic radiographs usually require two views taken at right angles to each other. These are called orthogonal views.

Gastrointestinal imaging studies

The commonest gastrointestinal (GI) contrast used is barium sulphate, which is completely inert but absorbs radiation very effectively. Different physical preparations of barium are used and in different concentrations depending on the study type, e.g. spherical molecules, considerably diluted, for small bowel studies, and small spikes of highly concentrated barium for upper GI studies. These latter molecules adhere to the oesophageal and gastric mucosa, allowing excellent mucosal definition, particularly if used with an effervescent, gas-producing powder (barium meal) or insufflated air (e.g. barium enema).

On occasion, e.g. if a gastrointestinal perforation is suspected, water-soluble contrast such as gastrograffin or iopamidol is used. This is because barium within the mediastinal space or peritoneal cavity is highly toxic, unlike the water-soluble media. They do, however, lack fine detail resolution and their role is chiefly to exclude obstruction and perforation.

Urography

Low osmolar water-soluble contrast such as iopamidol is injected intravenously and is filtered by the renal glomeruli, accumulating in the renal collecting system, and thus outlining it. Static images are taken to demonstrate the early 'nephrogram' phase, and the later pyelographic phase, when the renal calyces, pelvis, ureters and bladder are filled.

As in all forms of contrast radiology, the control film (Fig. 22.16), i.e. the film obtained prior to contrast administration, can provide valuable additional information (Fig. 22.16), e.g. presence of a subtle renal calculus, and should always be carefully reviewed.

Computed tomography

Like conventional radiography, computed tomography (CT) produces its images by generating x-ray photons. However, instead of a single x-ray screen/film, multiple detectors and the x-ray tube rotate inside the ring (gantry), which surrounds the patient. Modern scanners use a helical technique whereby the patient advances through the gantry as it rotates, acquiring a volume of data. Ultrafast, helical multidetector (multislice) CT scanners allow very rapid scanning of body areas (e.g. thorax in 10 seconds). Multiplanar reconstructions allow superb three-dimensional images to be created.

The CT image is divided into picture elements (pixels) corresponding to a block of tissue (voxel) within the patient. Each pixel has an attenuation value (shade of grey) which depends on the corresponding voxel's composition. The attenuation value is measured in 'Hounsfield units' (HU). Air is typically −1000 HU; fat −50 HU; water 0 HU; soft tissue 30–80 HU; and bone +500 HU (Fig. 16.5). Metallic implants are +1000 HU.

It is important to remember that the radiation dose to the patient following CT scanning is

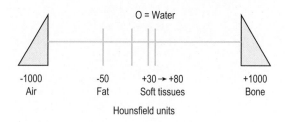

Fig. 16.5 Attenuation values on CT.

considerable. For instance, helical CT of the chest produces a radiation dose of about 400 chest x-rays!

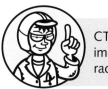

CT accounts for 4% of imaging but 40% of medical radiation exposure.

Interventional radiology

This now comprises a very significant component of medical imaging, and spans the disciplines of diagnosis and therapy. Interventional procedures cover a wide spectrum. They can be divided into those procedures that access a vessel or tube (e.g. cerebro- or cardiovascular, biliary or urological) and those that access a pathological lesion directly via the shortest percutaneous route (e.g. abscess drainage, tumour or nodal biopsy).

Those procedures that access a vessel or tube employ the modified Seldinger technique. Following initial puncture of the vessel with a needle, a guide wire is advanced along the lumen. The needle is withdrawn and a catheter advanced over the wire. Following correct catheter placement, subsequent delivery of angioplasty balloons, expandable stents, occluding coils, glues or microspheres are all feasible.

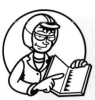

- List non-ionizing radiation imaging modalities.
- What factors must be considered when technically assessing the quality of a chest x-ray?
- What are orthogonal views?
- What is a Hounsfield unit?
- List the review areas on a chest x-ray assessment.
- Explain the modified Seldinger technique.

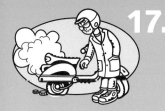

17. Non-ionizing Radiation Techniques

Ultrasound

Ultrasound has no ionizing radiation associated with it and there are no practical safety aspects within the diagnostic power range. Diagnostic ultrasound waves are produced by using an electromagnetic field to produce alteration of the physical shape of piezoelectric crystals (a transducer) within the probe. This shape alteration causes emission of the sound waves. These high frequency waves, having been emitted by the probe, enter the body, are reflected back by internal structures and are detected by the same probe. The diagnostic frequency range is between 2 and 20 MHz. Various probes of different frequencies are available depending on the structures being imaged.

The scanned region is represented on a monitor screen by shades of grey, the shade describing the tissue's echogenicity. Fatty tissue is slightly brighter (hyperechoic) than surrounding tissue, while fluid is completely black (anechoic). In modern real-time ultrasound machines, multiple transducer elements are arranged in rows (arrays) within the probe. These allow an instantaneous image that can be updated by altering the frame rate, usually a range of between 20 and 200 frames per second. Ultrasound is a dynamic investigation and observing the moving image is often more valuable than evaluating the static printed scans.

Ultrasound cannot penetrate gas or bone. Overlying ribs and aerated lung therefore prevent imaging of deeper structures.

Doppler ultrasound

The Doppler effect describes alteration in sound frequency caused by movement between the sound source and the observer, e.g. the changing pitch of a motorcycle engine as it passes a stationary spectator. In ultrasound, the sound source (and 'listener') is the probe. A dual function probe transducer produces what is known as 'pulsed wave Doppler'. Approximately 95% of the probe time is in the listening mode.

Movement of red blood cells relative to the probe produces alteration in frequency. This frequency change can be displayed as a spectral trace, a colour or an audible signal.

Common indications for Doppler ultrasound would include peripheral vascular examinations, particularly in lower limb diagnosis of deep venous thrombosis and venous insufficiency. Other indications include carotid Doppler examination in TIA/stroke/neurological disturbance, abdominal Doppler imaging in portal hypertension, Budd–Chiari syndrome and fetal–maternal medicine imaging of the umbilical vessels.

Abdominal ultrasound scan

Indications include abdominal pain, jaundice, renal dysfunction or obstruction, abdominal mass or abdominal distension.

What to look for

Ultrasound examination of the abdomen and pelvis is a methodical examination of the gallbladder, biliary tree, liver, spleen, pancreas, kidneys, aorta, vena cava and urinary bladder, and, in the female patient, the adnexa, i.e. the uterus, cervix and ovaries.

Patients referred for hepatobiliary ultrasound should be fasted for at least 4 hours. Those requiring pelvic ultrasound should have a full bladder.

Cardiac ultrasound

Echocardiography uses both a real-time image and M (movement) mode ultrasound. M mode ultrasound is a continuously moving amplitude (A mode) waveform. In A mode, the height of the 'spike' relates to its echointensity, and its position on the horizontal axis, its depth (like sonar).

Cardiac ultrasound is used to assess the heart chamber size, valve and wall motion. Common indications would be valve disease, septal defects, cardiomyopathy, cardiac failure, assessment of systolic function and quantification of pericardial effusion.

Magnetic resonance imaging

The physics of magnetic resonance (MR) depend on the fact that the nucleus of every hydrogen atom in every water molecule has magnetic properties. This is because they are charged particles, protons, which spin. If an external magnetic field is applied, these protons align themselves to that field, wobbling about the field axis with a motion known as 'precession'. When a second magnetic field, in the form of a radiofrequency (RF) pulse, is applied at right angles to the first, the protons' vector alters to become perpendicular to the external magnetic field, and they gain energy and spin synchronously. This is known as being 'in phase'.

Once the RF pulse stops, the protons do two things: firstly they shed their extra newly acquired energy back to the surrounding chemical lattice. This is known as T1 relaxation. Secondly, they stop spinning synchronously. This asynchronous dephasing is known as T2 relaxation.

As a rule, T1 images produce good anatomical detail, whereas T2 images are more representative of tissue pathology. Inversion recovery (IR) or fat suppression sequences highlight areas of fluid, both normal (e.g. CSF) and pathological (e.g. focal areas of infection, trauma, inflammation and malignancy).

MRI was initially used for the evaluation of the central nervous system, i.e. the brain and spinal cord (see Fig. 24.1). More recently multiple and diverse applications of MRI have been realized. In neuroradiological imaging, perfusion and diffusion imaging has evolved in the evaluation of strokes and of focal brain lesions and tumour recurrence, respectively. Improved resolution and faster imaging times have resulted in MR being used to image the biliary tree (magnetic resonance cholangiopancreatography, MRCP), and the central and peripheral vascular systems (magnetic resonance angiography, MRA).

- When might Doppler ultrasound be used?
- What patient preparation might be necessary before ultrasound of the abdomen?
- What is the difference between T1 and T2 weighted MR imaging?
- What should be checked with a patient before undergoing an MRI scan?

18. Nuclear Medicine

Nuclear medicine is a specialty that produces images of function rather than anatomy. Tiny amounts of radiopharmaceuticals (usually of the order of micrograms) permit imaging without interference in the body's physiological and biochemical processes. Radiopharmaceuticals are labelled with radioactive isotopes which decay to produce gamma photons (like high energy x-rays).

Different types of gamma camera are used to detect these gamma photons and produce an image of the radiopharmaceutical distribution within the body. Many different radiopharmaceuticals and radioisotopes are utilized to image different functions in various body organs.

The quantity (dose) of radiopharmaceutical used is measured in megaBecquerels or MBq (1 Becquerel is one decay per second). The dose is a balance between image quality, from lots of gamma photons, and minimum radiation effects within the patient.

Average UK annual background radiation is 2.2 mSV.

Nuclear imaging produces functional rather than structural images.

The amount of radiation absorbed by the patient is called the effective dose (ED) and is measured in milliSieverts (mSv). Generally, the longer the half-life of a radioisotope, the higher its ED.

Conventions

Isotopes are described by their atomic weight, e.g. Tc^{99m} (technetium). Doses are given as megaBecquerels (MBq) and the effective dose (ED) as milliSieverts (mSv).

$Technetium^{99m}$ is the most common radioisotope used in nuclear medicine because of its characteristics. The short (6 hour) half-life allows labelling of the radiopharmaceutical, transfer to the imaging department, injection of the patient and imaging, but within 24 hours very little radioactivity is present in the patient (Fig. 18.1). Gamma photons of a specific and single energy level are produced and are detected by the gamma camera.

$Indium^{111}$ is usually used when images need to be obtained beyond 24 hours. This is important if uptake of the radiopharmaceutical is slow or if the function being imaged is intermittent. This may be used for the detection of an abscess or in assessing the extent and distribution of inflammatory bowel disease using radiolabelled white cells.

$Iodine^{123}$ is often used when new pharmaceuticals are produced because the chemistry of labelling compounds with iodine is often simpler.

Single photon emission computed tomography (SPECT)

Radioactive decay from tissues surrounding the organ of interest can reduce the image contrast, and activity in adjacent viscera or blood vessels reduces the ability to quantify the core activity. Tomography addresses both these issues. In single photon emission computed tomography (SPECT) studies, a conventional gamma camera rotates 360° around the patient. Standard isotopes such as technetium are used. A single photon from each nuclear disintegration is identified.

Positron emission tomography (PET)

Positron emission tomography (PET) is a relatively new and rapidly expanding nuclear medicine

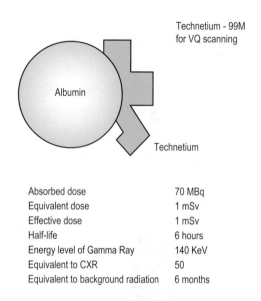

Technetium - 99M
for VQ scanning

Absorbed dose	70 MBq
Equivalent dose	1 mSv
Effective dose	1 mSv
Half-life	6 hours
Energy level of Gamma Ray	140 KeV
Equivalent to CXR	50
Equivalent to background radiation	6 months

Fig. 18.1 Typical radioisotope.

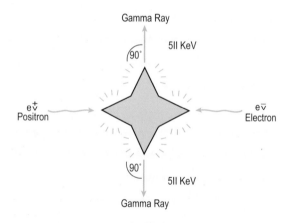

Fig. 18.2 Positron emission tomography annihilation event.

technique which utilizes the emission of positrons by specific isotopes. Such elements contain excess protons that decay to form a neutron and a positron (antimatter). A positron is a positively charged electron. The positron travels approximately 2 mm beyond the atom and collides with an electron. The collision, known as annihilation, results in the formation of two gamma rays with a specific energy of 511 keV (Fig. 18.2). These two gamma rays travel in opposite directions

and are absorbed by two detectors located around the patient. The PET scanner's computer system can subsequently localize the site of the annihilation event within the patient.

The most frequently used isotope in clinical practice is fluorodeoxyglucose[18] (FDG). This radiopharmaceutical images glucose uptake via glucose transporter proteins. These are overexpressed in most common malignancies. Such tumours are said to be 'glucose avid' and absorb the glucose analogue, FDG. When subsequent positron emission begins within the tumour, detectors localize its position within the body. It is therefore possible to identify sites of active or recurrent disease, and to differentiate them from scar tissue or fibrosis. The disadvantages of PET are that not all tumours are glucose avid, the isotopes are short lived (FDG, 2 hours) and a cyclotron is required to produce them.

PET–CT combines PET (functional imaging) with CT (structural imaging) to give the best results.

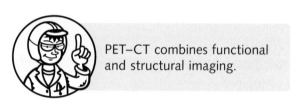

PET–CT combines functional and structural imaging.

Specific isotope studies

Lung scanning (ventilation perfusion, V/Q scans)

Lung scanning is almost always performed to identify a pulmonary embolus (PE). An acute PE disrupts the blood supply to part of the lung without interfering with ventilation. Isotope scanning identifies this area which is ventilated but not perfused—a mismatch—and permits the diagnosis to be made. Segmental areas of absent perfusion with normal ventilation are seen in PE.

Perfusion scanning is performed with technetium labelled to macroaggregates of albumin (MAA). These have a diameter of 100 μm and image the perfusion at the pre-alveolar arteriolar level. The dose is 70 MBq (ED = 1 mSv).

Ventilation imaging may be performed with a variety of isotopes, e.g. krypton Kr^{81m}, eluted from a rubidium generator. The dose of krypton is 6000 MBq, but because the half-life is only 13 seconds, the ED is only 0.2 mSv. Alternatives include Xenon, Xe^{133} (400 MBq, ED = 0.4 mSv) or technetium labelled aerosols, e.g. DTPA (80 MBq, ED = 0.4 mSV). Note that the ED of all ventilation scans is very small.

Bone scanning

Bone scanning is performed with technetium methylene diphosphonate, $Tc^{99m}MDP$ (and other similar diphosphonates). The dose is 555 MBq and the ED is 1 mSv. This radiopharmaceutical images osteoblastic activity and the deposition of hydroxyapatite into the osteoid matrix.

There are two chief forms of bone scanning: static and dynamic. With static studies, images are acquired 2 hours after IV administration. This is principally performed to stage malignancy, establish the presence of fractures or identify metabolic bone disease. In dynamic studies, images are acquired immediately at the time of injection (flow phase), 5–10 minutes later (pool phase) and at the 2 hour (static) phase. This type of bone scan is used to establish the presence of osteomyelitis.

Kidney
Renal structure

This is evaluated (as is renal function) using a technetium labelled DMSA (dimercaptosuccinic acid) scan. The dose is 80 MBq and the ED is 1.0 mSv. This radiopharmaceutical images the amount of functioning proximal convoluted tubular cells and is used to image acute and chronic pyelonephritis. This allows for assessment of differential renal function.

Renal excretion

There is a choice of two isotopes: Tc-labelled MAG-3 (mercaptoacetyltriglycene) which is actively excreted at the proximal convoluted tubule, or DTPA (diethylene triamine pentacetic acid) which is filtered at the glomerulus. ED is 0.7 mSv. These scans assess how efficiently the urine produced by the kidney drains into the ureter and bladder.

Thyroid scanning

Thyroid studies image the function of the sodium–iodide symporter chain. The isotope chiefly used in imaging the thyroid is technetium pertechnetate

$(Tc^{99m}O_4^-)$ with a dose of 80 MBq (ED = 1 mSv). Thyroid isotope studies can also be performed with an iodine isotope, I^{123}, with a dose of 20 MBq (ED = 3 mSv). Note that the effective dose is larger for I^{123} even though a smaller dose is given. This is because of its longer half-life.

Parathyroid scanning

Isotopes used are technetium pertechnetate, with a dose of 70 MBq, and Tc^{99m} MIBI (methoxyisobutyl isonitrile). MIBI is taken up by both the thyroid and the parathyroid adenoma whereas technetium is taken up by only the thyroid. As MIBI is not taken up by the normal parathyroid, it is possible to subtract one image from the other and localize parathyroid adenomas.

Lymphangiography

In this test, the transport of extracellular proteins through lymphatics of an affected limb is imaged. The isotope used is technetium human albumin nanocolloid. The dose is 40 MBq and the ED is 0.5 mSv. The study is typically performed to evaluate lower limb lymphatics. Isotope is injected into the web space between the toes. Inguinal nodes are imaged between 1 and 3 hours later, but in diseased states may be imaged at up to 24 hours.

Cardiac imaging

This test images the perfusion of the oxygenated functioning myocardial tissue and depends on the radiopharmaceutical (Tc^{99m} MIBI) being trapped in the functioning mitochondria. The dose is 400 MBq with an ED of 0.5 mSv.

Thallium (Tl^{201}), which was previously the traditionally used myocardial radiopharmaceutical, is a potassium analogue that images the perfusion of cardiac muscle with a functioning, energy-dependent Na/K ATPase system.

Myocardial perfusion imaging may help distinguish necrotic from ischaemic myocardium.

Adrenal medullary imaging

Adrenal imaging is performed with I^{123} MIBG (meta-iodo-benzyl-guanidine). This is a guanethidine analogue taken up by cells which produce adrenaline, e.g. adrenergic nerve cells and the adrenal medulla. The dose is 400 MBq with an ED of 6 mSv. This is used in the investigation of a phaeochromocytoma, in particular localization of extra-adrenal lesions.

White cell imaging

This can be performed with technetium HMPAO (Ceretec) with a dose of 200 MBq or with indium tropolone with a dose of 20–40 MBq (ED = 9 mSv). The radiopharmaceutical is used to label the patient's own white blood cells derived from a large (120 ml) blood sample which is subsequently reinjected. This scan images granulocyte migration from the intravascular to the extravascular space and is used to image infection and inflammatory bowel disease.

Red cell imaging

This is usually performed with technetium and sometimes indium labelled red cells. Red cell imaging identifies very small amounts of blood loss into the gastrointestinal tract. The camera detects movement of labelled red blood cells from the intravascular space into the gut lumen.

Blood loss is evaluated with images taken at 1, 2, 6 and 24 hours following the injection. The dose is 400 MBq. Technetium labelled sulphur colloid (dose 80 MBq) can also be used. Both techniques image active bleeding during the study and can detect a bleeding rate down to 0.5 ml per minute.

Liver and spleen imaging

Any colloid is useful; for example, technetium sulphur colloid, technetium antimony sulphide colloid and technetium tin colloid. Spleen imaging is with technetium labelled heat denatured red blood cells. Dose is 40 MBq with an ED of 2 mSv. These are now rarely used.

Biliary imaging

Biliary imaging is performed using technetium hepatoiminodiacetic acid (HIDA). The dose is 80–120 MBq with an ED of 1 mSv. The HIDA compounds image the drainage of bile from the liver, through the biliary tree and into the duodenum.

Chronic infection

This can be imaged with gallium (Ga^{67}). The dose is 150 MBq and the ED is 12 mSv. Ga^{67} is an iron analogue, and iron is a requirement of many bacteria. Gallium is also taken up by sarcoid and many tumours.

Tumour imaging

Octreotide is indium[111] labelled sandostatin. The dose is 185 MBq. The half life is 2–3 days. The octreotide images somatostatin receptors produced by many neuroendocrine tumours. Images are taken at 24 and 48 hours. It is useful in evaluating GI hormone tumours such as carcinoid, vipoma and insulinoma.

The principal radionuclides used in medical imaging are outlined in Figure 18.3.

Radiation doses and requests

Statutory regulations, namely the Ionizing Radiation Medical Exposure Regulations (IRMER) 2000, require referrers, practitioners and operators to limit the dose of diagnostic radiation to patients. Each exposure must be justified (Fig. 18.4).

The additional lifetime risk of acquiring a fatal cancer from the Earth's background radiation or a chest x-ray is 1 in a million. However, following an abdominal CT examination, the risk rises sharply to 1 in 2000. Conversely, the risk of acquiring a malignancy during one's lifetime is 1 in 3. Therefore the risk–benefit of an examination must always be considered. This is particularly pertinent if repeated imaging is required.

The Royal College of Radiologists has issued guidance for doctors in its booklet *Making the Best use of a Radiology Department* (5th edn, 2003). Reproduced below are two tables from this booklet (Figs 18.5, 18.6) illustrating the doses of common imaging investigations.

Principal radionuclides used in medical imaging

Element	Radionuclide	Half-life	Energy level	Use
Technetium	Tc^{99m}	6 hours	140 keV	Organ imaging
Gallium	Ga^{67}	7–8 hours	90–93 keV 185 keV 300 keV	Localization of neoplasms, abscesses and sarcoid
Krypton	Kr^{81m}	13.5 seconds	190 keV	Lung ventilation imaging
Indium	In^{111}	2.8 days	171 keV 250 keV	Cell labelling and CSF imaging, longer studies generally
Iodine	I^{123}	13.3 hours	160 keV	Use in thyroid and adrenal imaging (MIBG)
Iodine	I^{131}	8.1 days	610 keV 360 keV	Use in thyroid treatment (hyperthyroidism and thyroid cancer)
Thallium	Tl^{201}	74 hours	70 keV	Myocardial imaging

Fig. 18.3 Principal radionuclides used in medical imaging.

Attach addressograph Label or print in CAPITALS

Hospital No: _____ BR 645268 _____

Full Name: _____

Address: _____

_____

DOB: 22 / 11 / 54   Tel No: _____

Ward/Dept: 6F   Consultant: WEEKLEY

Departmental Use Only

ID Check

Name ☐

Address ☐

DOB ☐

Date of Appointment: _____

Time: _____ Room No: _____

Pregnancy Status (delete as applicable)
Pregnant / Not Pregnant **LMP** / /
Breast feeding: Yes / No

Summary of clinical history (50) 25 year-history Rheumatoid disease. Two years on Methotrexate. No previous chest disease 6/12 ↑ SOB, dry cough. Exercise tolerance 100 yards o/E Bilateral basal fine inspiratory crepitations

Mobility Status
Bed ☑ Portable ☐
Walking ☐ Chair ☐

What clinical queries should this study answer?
Interstitial lung Disease?

Infection Status
MRSA ⊕

Pressure Risk Score
NO RISK

For specialist examinations, please state known contra-indiations.
Nil Contraindication

Patient Category
NHS ☑   Private ☐   Category 2 ☐

All previous images must accompany patients.

Examination suggested: HRCT CHEST

Pregnant: Yes / No N/A
LMP / /

REFERRER:

Referrer (signature) _____ Name (printed) _____

Job title: CONS/SPR/SHO/JHO/NP/GP (please circle) Bleep/Contact No. 2064   Date 24/11/2004

All incomplete and illegible forms will be returned.

Fig. 18.4 X-ray request.

Typical effective doses from diagnostic medical exposure in the 2000s

Diagnostic procedure	Typical effective doses (mSv)	Equivalent no. of chest x-rays	Equivalent period of background radiation
Limb/joint except hip	<0.01	<0.5	<1.5 days
Chest (PA film)	0.02	1	3 days
Skull	0.06	3	9 days
Thoracic spine	0.07	35	4 months
Lumbar spine	1.0	50	5 months
Hip	0.4	20	2 months
Pelvis	0.7	35	4 months
Abdomen	0.7	35	4 months
IVU	2.4	120	14 months
Barium swallow	1.5	75	8 months
Barium meal	2.6	130	15 months
Barium follow-through	3	150	16 months
Barium enema	7.2	360	3.2 years
CT head	2.0	100	10 months
CT chest	8	400	3.6 years
CT abdomen or pelvis	10	500	4.5 years
Lung ventilation (Xe^{133})	0.3	15	7 weeks
Lung perfusion (Tc^{99m})	1	50	6 months
Kidney (Tc^{99m})	1	50	6 months
Thyroid (Tc^{99m})	1	50	6 months
Bone (Tc^{99m})	4	200	1.8 years
Dynamic cardiac (Tc^{99m})	6	300	2.7 years
PET head (^{18}FDG)	5	250	2.3 years

Fig. 18.5 Typical effective doses from diagnostic medical exposure in the 2000s. (Reproduced with permission from the Royal College of Radiologists.)

Band classification of the typical effective doses of ionizing radiation from common imaging procedures

Band	Typical effective dose (mSv)	Examples
0	0	US, MRI
I	<1	CXR, XR limb, XR pelvis
II	1–5	IVU, XR lumbar spine, NM (e.g. skeletal scintigram), CT head and neck
III	6–10	CT chest or abdomen, NM (e.g. cardiac)
IV	>10	Extensive CT studies, some NM studies (e.g. PET)

Fig. 18.6 Band classification of the typical effective doses of ionizing radiation from common imaging procedures. (Reproduced with permission from the Royal College of Radiologists.)

Always consider radiation dose when requesting imaging investigations.

- In what unit is a radiopharmaceutical dose measured?
- What properties make technetium^{99m} a good radioisotope for clinical imaging?
- When might PET imaging be useful?
- What regulations govern the use of radiation in patients?
- What is the effective dose of a CT chest?

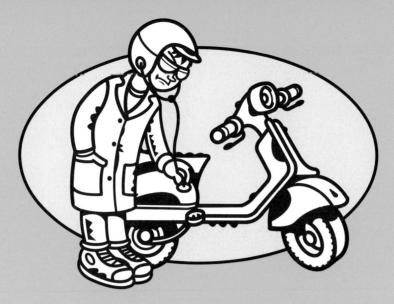

IMAGE GALLERY

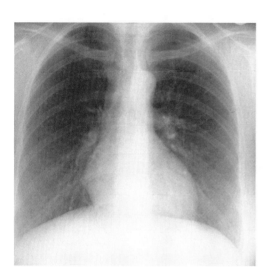

Fig. 19.1 Reference chest x-ray (CXR). All areas to be assessed.
- patient details
- technical factors
- cardiac silhouette
- mediastinum
- lungs
- bones
- soft tissues

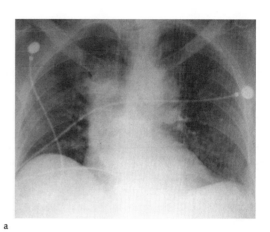

a

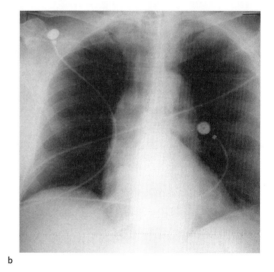

b

Fig. 19.2 Normal CXR: (a) Poor inspiratory effort; (b) the same patient with normal inspiratory effort.

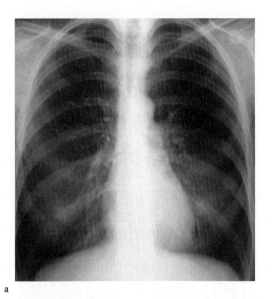

a

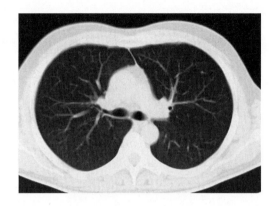

Fig. 19.4 CT chest: Section at the level of the right upper lobe bronchus (RULB).

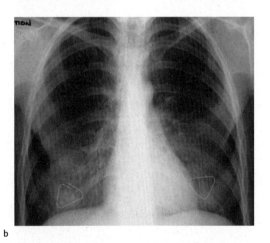

b

Fig. 19.3. Female CXR: (a) With nipple shadows; (b) with nipple markers, showing their usefulness. These are used to differentiate nipple shadows from an intrapulmonary mass.

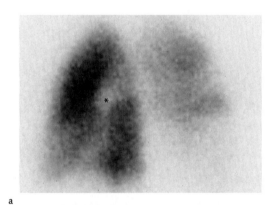

a

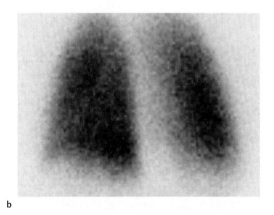

b

Fig. 19.5 VQ Scan: Pulmonary emboli. (a) Lung perfusion (b) lung ventilation. There are perfusion defects (*); ventilation scan normal, unmatched defect .

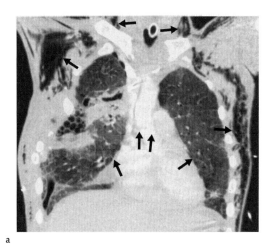

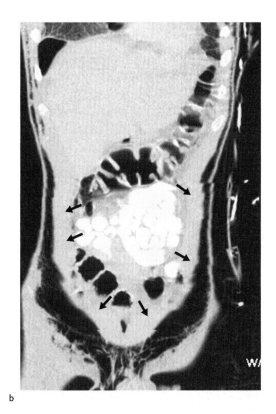

a

b

Fig. 19.6 Surgical emphysema in polytrauma, CT scan: (a) chest; (b) abdomen. Air in the soft tissues (arrows) extends from the neck to the scrotum.

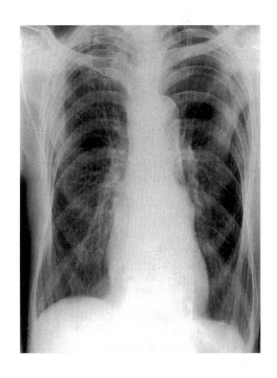

Fig. 19.7 Emphysema, CXR: Lungs overinflated • Greater than 10 ribs visible posteriorly • Flattened diaphragms • Enlarged central pulmonary arteries • Peripheral pruning.

107

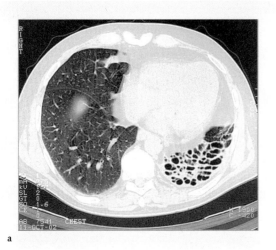

a

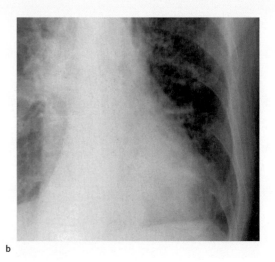

b

Fig. 19.8 Bronchiectasis, (a) high-resolution CT scan, (b) CXR left lower lobe: Enlarged bronchi with crowding • Bronchi visible to the extremity of lung field • May be fluid levels within the bronchi • May be associated consolidation • May be associated interstitial lung disease.

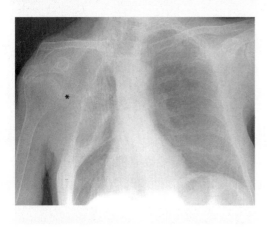

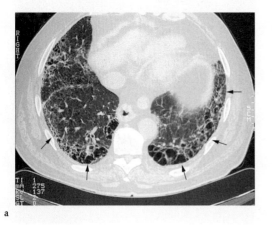

Fig. 19.9 Right apical tuberculosis, previous thoracoplasty, CXR (*): Increased density • Scarring • Interstitial lung changes and volume loss.

a

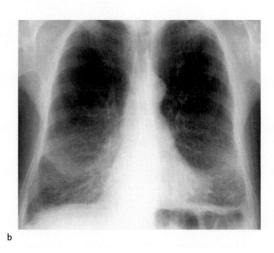

b

Fig. 19.10 Bilateral pulmonary fibrosis, (a) high-resolution CT scan, (b) CXR: Subpleural location and basal predominance • Reticulonodular shadowing ('lines and dots' appearance) • Cardiac and diaphragmatic silhouette may be visible on x-ray.

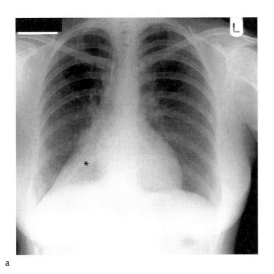
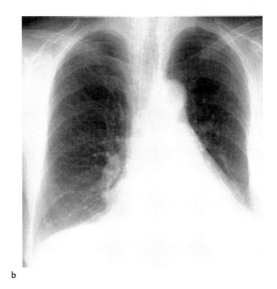

Fig. 19.11 **Lower lobe consolidation, CXR**: (a) Right lower lobe (*); (b) left lower lobe. Loss of the right/left hemidiaphragm • Elevation of the diaphragm • Ipsilateral mediastinal shift.

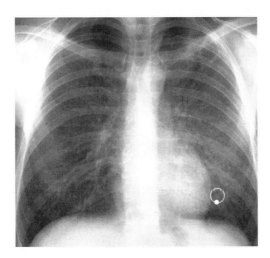

Fig. 19.12 *Pneumocystis jiroveci* (formerly *P. carinii*) **pneumonia, CXR**: Initial interstitial pattern • Progression to air space change within 5 days • There are subtle perihilar interstitial markings that will progress, if untreated, to form consolidation.

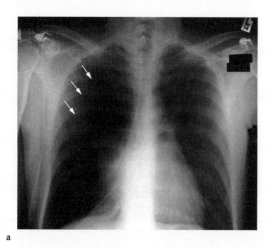

a

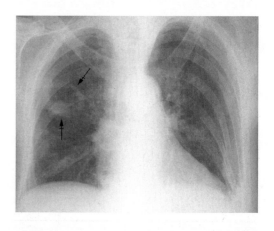

Fig. 19.14 Cavitating right lung, CXR: Opacity seen within the lung • Central lucency within opacity, plus or minus fluid level.

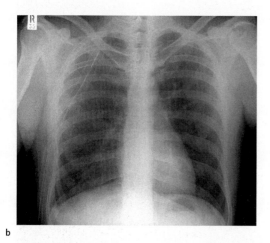

b

Fig. 19.13 Pneumothorax, CXR: (a) Right side pre-drain; (b) chest drain in place. Note difference in transradiancy (blackess) between the two pre-drain lungs • Pre-drain collapsed lung edge identifiable (arrows) with tension, depression of diaphragm and contralateral mediastinal shift • Post-drain no lung edge visible, mediastinum and diaphragm in normal position.

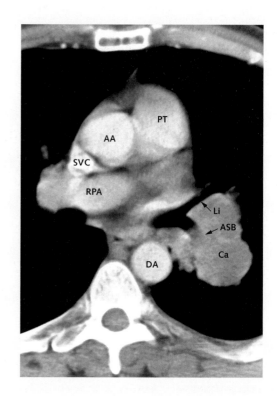

Fig. 19.15 Carcinoma of left lung, CT scan: Low attenuation mass adjacent to hilum, endobronchial compression, associated lymphadenopathy. (AA, ascending aorta; ASB, apical segmental; bronchus of the left lower lobe; Ca, carcinoma of the left lung; DA, descending aorta; Li, lingular bronchus; PT, pulmonary trunk; RPA, right pulmonary artery; SVC, superior vena cava.)

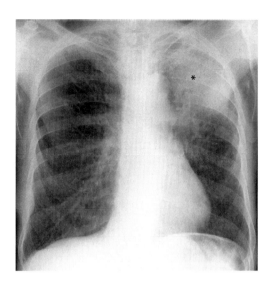

Fig. 19.16 Left apical carcinoma, CXR: Increased-density apex (*) • Irregular margin, does not correspond to lobe • May be bulging of associated fissures • May be associated lymphadenopathy or metastatic disease • Associated rib erosion.

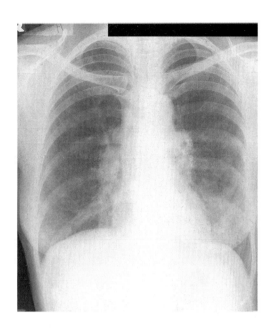

Fig. 19.18 Sarcoidosis, CXR: Bilateral hilar lymphadenopathy • May be right paratracheal lymphadenopathy (Garland's syndrome) • Look for interstitial lung disease.

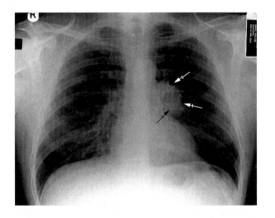

Fig. 19.17 Left hilar mass, CXR: Enlarged left hilum • May be associated consolidation and volume loss • Look for central lymphadenopathy • Look for pulmonary metastases • The hila, although at different levels, should normally be the same size and density.

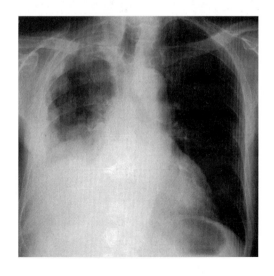

Fig. 19.19 Right sided mesothelioma, CXR: Nobulated pleural thickening with lobulated nature • Lesion encircles right lung • No volume loss.

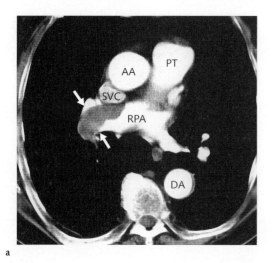

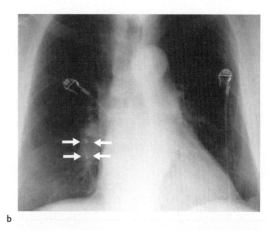

Fig. 19.20 Pulmonary embolus, (a) contrast-enhanced CT, (b) CXR: Large embolus seen within right pulmonary artery (arrows) • Enlarged right pulmonary artery. (DA, descending aorta; AA, ascending aorta; SVC, superior vena cava; RPA, right pulmonary artery; PT, pulmonary trunk.

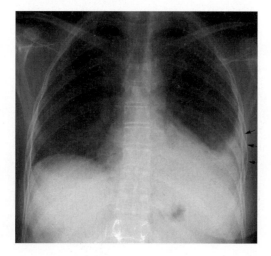

Fig. 19.21 Left pleural effusion, erect CXR: Loss of left hemidiaphragm • Meniscus laterally at chest wall (arrows) • Lack of mediastinal movement indicates associated underlying lobe or collapse.

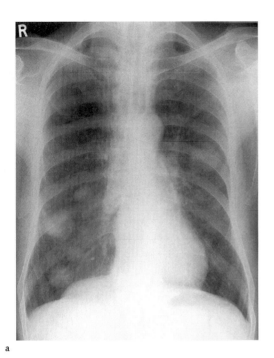

a

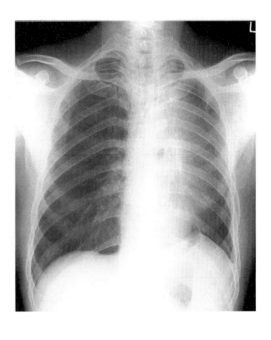

Fig. 19.23 Left upper lobe collapse, CXR: Decreased visibility of aortic knuckle, veil-like opacity, diaphragmatic elevation and ipsilateral mediastinal elevation.

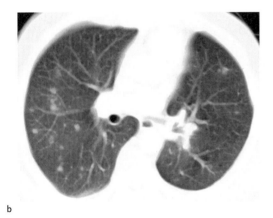

b

Fig. 19.22 Pulmonary metastases, (a) CXR, (b) CT: Multiple pulmonary nodules evident • Non-specific appearance • Patient history essential.

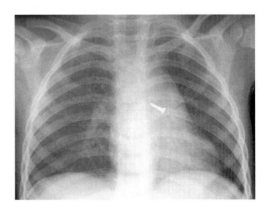

Fig. 19.24 Inhaled foreign body in left main bronchus, CXR: Foreign body may be visible • Initially overinflation of lung with diaphragmatic depression and contralateral mediastinal movement; later there is volume loss, diaphragmatic elevation and ipsilateral mediastinal movement.

113

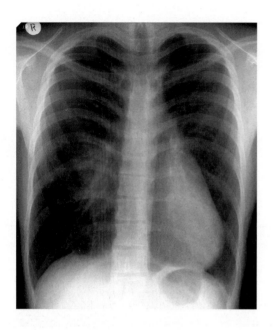

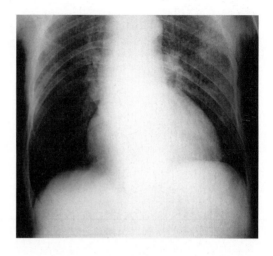

Fig. 19.26 Miliary tuberculosis, CXR: Fine opacities within both lungs • Appearance is non-specific so patient history essential.

Fig. 19.25 Pectus excavatum, CXR: Cardiac silhouette displaces to the left, mimicking right middle lobe consolidation, heart shaped ribs • Diagnosis is confirmed by examining patient (not by performing lateral CXR).

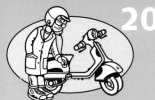
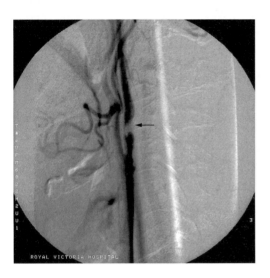

Fig. 20.1 Internal carotid artery, carotid angiogram:
Area of stenosis identified beyond the bifurcation of the
carotid artery • Distal carotid vessel patent • External
carotid artery patent.

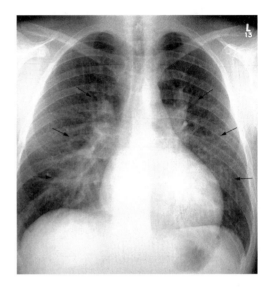

Fig. 20.3 Atrial septal defect, CXR: Pulmonary plethora
± cardiomegaly • Small aortic knuckle • Aortic knuckle
contour may or may not be normal.

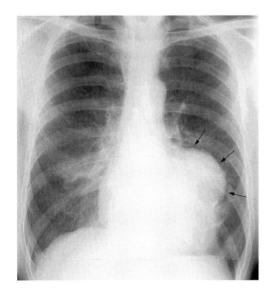

Fig. 20.2 Left ventricular aneurysm, chest x-ray (CXR):
Square shape to left ventricle (arrows) • May be
cardiomegaly • Look for evidence of cardiac failure •
May be ventricular calcification.

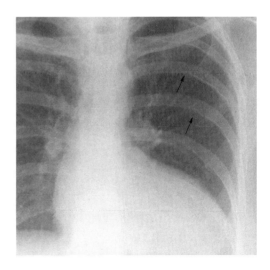

Fig. 20.4 Aortic coarctation, CXR: Notching identified
ribs 4–10 (Dock's sign, arrows).

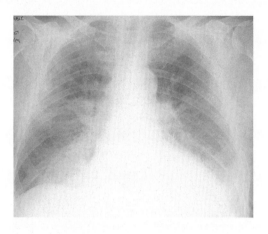

Fig. 20.5 Cardiac failure, CXR: The heart is enlarged • Increased pulmonary venous vascularity • Upper zone diversion • Kerley B lines • Pleural effusions • Air space consolidation in pulmonary oedema.

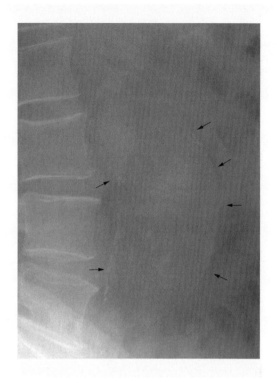

Fig. 20.7 Abdominal aortic aneurysm (arrows), lateral lumbar spine x-ray: Calcification of the aorta • Loss of aortic wall parallelism • Superior mesenteric artery if calcified provides good marker for the position of renal arteries.

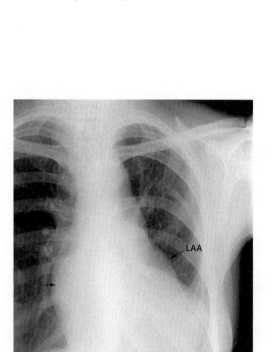

Fig. 20.6 Left atrial enlargement, CXR: Cardiomegaly • Splaying of the carina (angle greater than 90°) • Left atrial appendage (LAA) enlargement (arrow) • Double atrial shadow • In this case the left atrial wall is calcified.

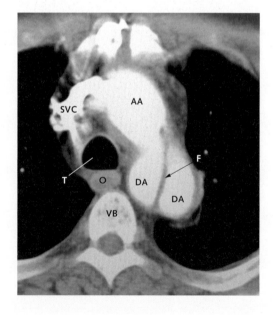

Fig. 20.8 Aortic dissection, CT chest. (AA, ascending aortic arch; DA, descending aortic arch; F, dissection flap; O, oesophagus; SVC, superior vena cava; T, trachea; VB, vertebral body.)

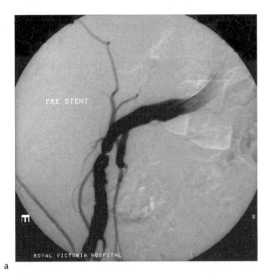

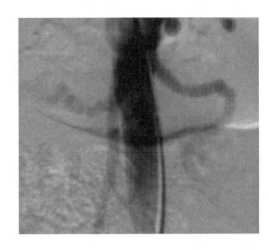

Fig. 20.10 Fibromuscular hyperplasia, renal artery angiogram: Beaded appearance to renal arteries.

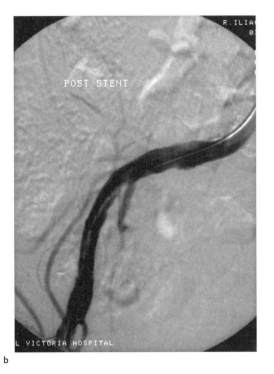

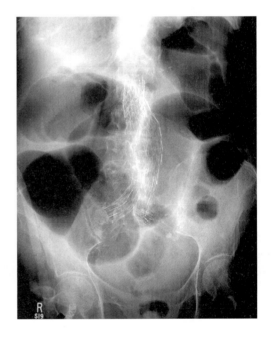

Fig. 20.9 Right iliac artery, DSA: Pre-intervention irregularity and narrowing of the right external iliac artery • Post-intervention diameter of vessel restored • No significant stenosis • Check distal vessels remain patent • The radiologist will check no residual pressure gradient across the stent.

Fig. 20.11 Aortic stent placement, AXR: Stent appearance will vary according to manufacturer • Typically metallic lattice along the length of the aortic ± iliac arteries.

117

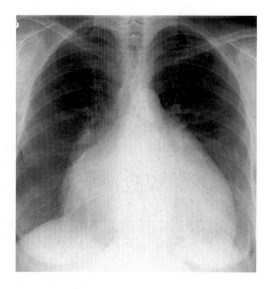

Fig. 20.12 Pericardial effusion, CXR: Heart significantly enlarged and has globular appearance • Diagnosis confirmed on echocardiography.

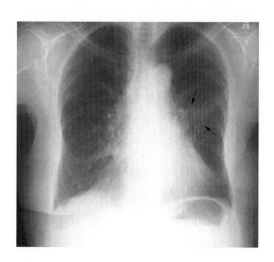

Fig. 20.14 CT abdomen: Inferior vena caval filter (arrows).

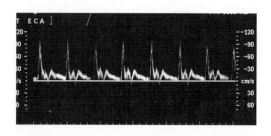

Fig. 20.13 Doppler spectral waveform: Normal external carotid artery.

Fig. 20.15 Left mastectomy, CXR: Different transparency of both lungs • Left breast shadow absent • Left hilar mass (arrows). Indicates recurrent disease.

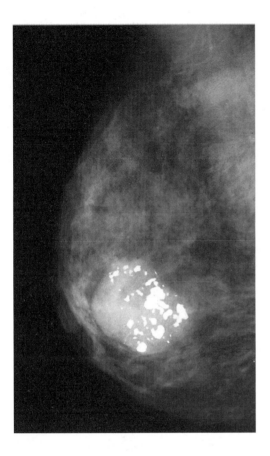

Fig. 20.16 Mammogram, oblique view: Fibroadenoma with popcorn calcification.

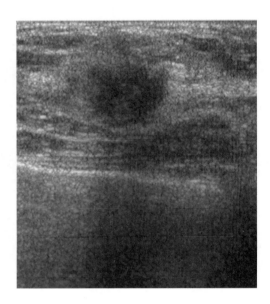

Fig. 20.17 Ultrasound: Breast carcinoma.

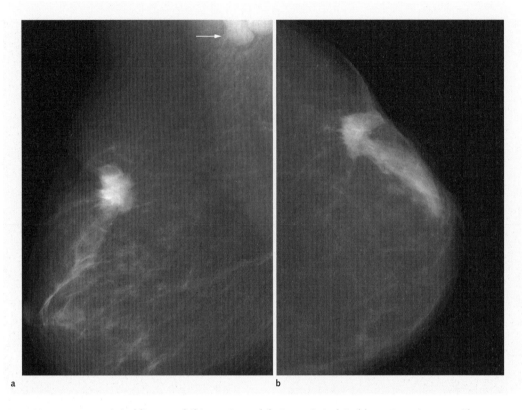

Fig. 20.18 Mammograms, (a) oblique and (b) craniocaudal views: Spiculated breast carcinoma with lymphadenopathy and skin retraction.

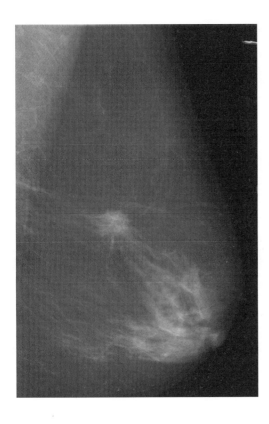

Fig. 20.19 Mammogram, oblique view: Spiculated breast carcinoma.

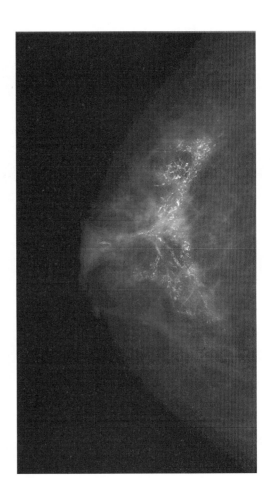

Fig. 20.21 Mammogram, craniocaudal view: Branching calcification in keeping with carcinoma.

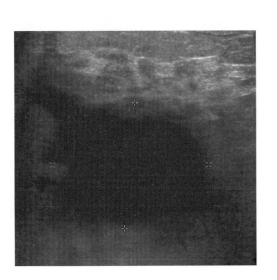

Fig. 20.20 Ultrasound: Breast abscess.

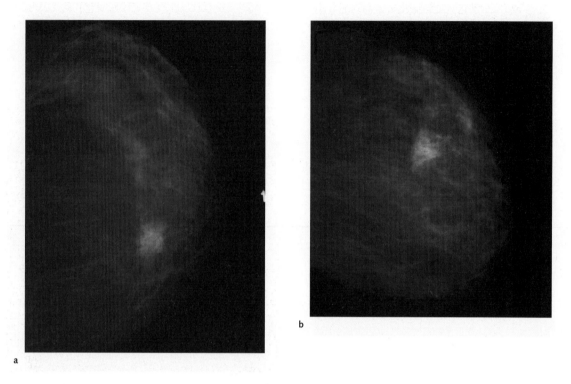

Fig. 20.22 Mammograms, (a) oblique and (b) craniocaudal views: Spiculated mass in keeping with a carcinoma.

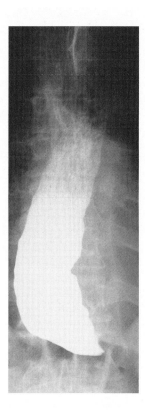

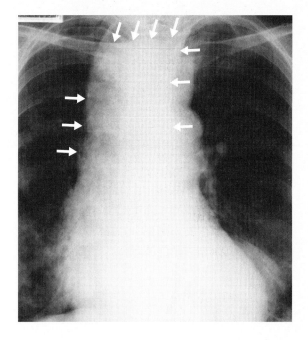

Fig. 21.2 Achalasia, chest x-ray (CXR): Grossly widened mediastinum (arrows) • Distended, fluid-filled oesophagus is seen in the midline (arrows), extending into the neck • Extends above level of aortic knuckle • Fluid level may be apparent • Signs of chronic aspiration may be apparent in lower lobes of lung • Typically a small gastric shadow on chest x-ray.

Fig. 21.1 Achalasia, barium swallow: Dilated oesophagus • Smooth contour to walls • Tapers to a beak at distal end • No shouldering of oesophageal lesion.

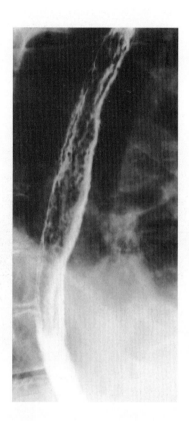

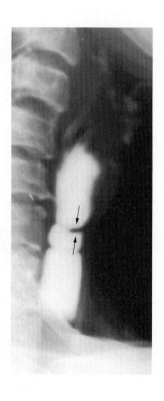

Fig. 21.3 Candidiasis, barium swallow: Multiple small filling defects • Irregular mucosa • Long segment involvement (continuous).

Fig. 21.4 Oesophageal web, barium swallow: Usually situated at pharyngo-oesophageal junction (C6 vertebra) • Thin, linear filling defect • Normally arises from anterior oesophageal wall • Can be circumferential and multiple • In association with iron deficiency anaemia and koilonychia known as Paterson–Brown Kelly (Plummer–Vinson) syndrome • Risk of development of oesophageal malignancy.

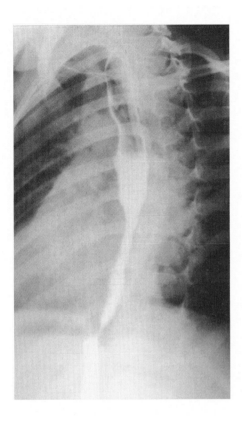

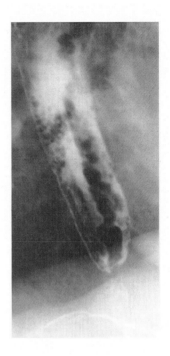

Fig. 21.6 Oesophageal varices, barium swallow:
Multiple • Long serpiginous filling defects.

Fig. 21.5 Corrosive (benign) stricture, barium swallow:
Long segment involvement • Smooth contour to
stricture when established (after acute incident) • Often
proximal dilatation of oesophagus • With time may
develop oesophageal malignancy (see Fig. 21.7 for
features) • Commonly occurs in children from accidental
ingestion of corrosive liquid.

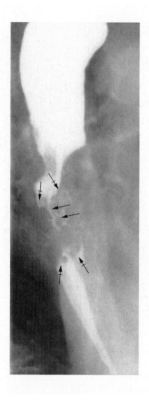

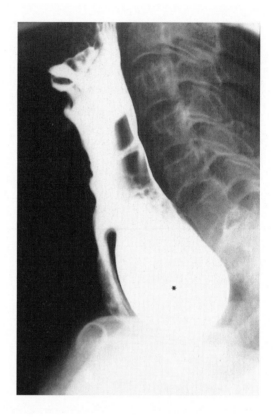

Fig. 21.7 Oesophageal carcinoma, barium swallow:
Short stricture • Loss of normal mucosa giving an
irregular outline—note the shouldered margins of the
tumour (barred arrows) and the irregular, narrowed
mucosa (arrows) • With an irregular mucosa is the key
finding of malignancy • Short shouldered lesion.

Fig. 21.8 Pharyngeal pouch, barium swallow: Pooling
of barium in pharyngeal outpouching (*) • Occurs at
Killian's dehiscence • Relative contraindication for
endoscopy in 'dysphagia' patient • Disease of older
patients (>55 years of age).

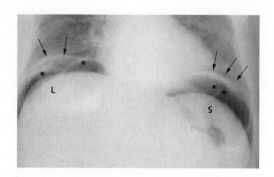

Fig. 21.9 Pneumoperitoneum, erect CXR: Free air (*) under both hemidiaphragms (arrows) (L, liver; S, spleen) •
Usually more on the right, interposed between the diaphragm and liver • Gastric 'air' bubble may obscure on
the left side and may be mistaken for free air.

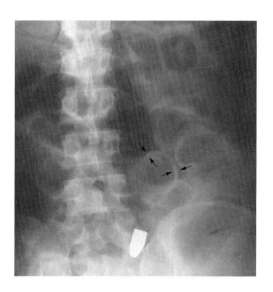

Fig. 21.10 Pneumoperitoneum, Rigler's sign, supine CXR: The bowel wall is visible (arrows), because of gas within bowel lumen and peritoneum, latter seen as air within the fibres of the psoas muscle • Pneumoperitoneum due to a gun-shot wound.

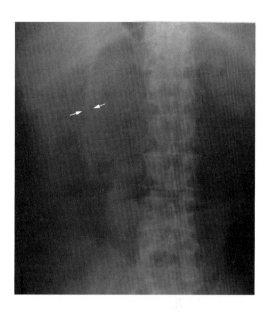

Fig. 21.11 Pneumoperitoneum falciform ligament sign, supine abdominal x-ray (AXR): Falciform ligament outlined by free gas (arrows) • Extends from liver to umbilicus (umbilicus relates to L3).

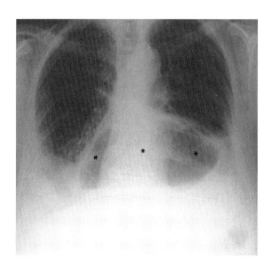

Fig. 21.12 Hiatus hernia, retrocardiac air-fluid level, CXR: Mediastinal soft tissue mass (*) • Left lateral film will confirm the retrocardiac level • Barium study will confirm the diagnosis.

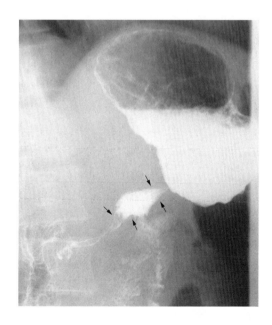

Fig. 21.13 Gastric carcinoma, barium meal: Irregular appearance to mucosa • Contracted lumen of stomach • Differential diagnosis of a gastric lymphoma should be considered.

127

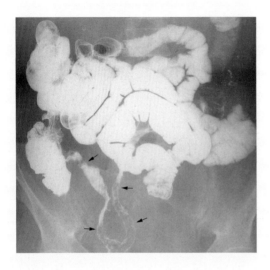

Fig. 21.14 Crohn's disease string sign (of Kantor), small bowel study: There is a well-defined strictured segment of small bowel in the ileum (arrows)—may be short, long, single or multiple • Rose thorn ulceration (due to deep fissured ulceration) • Bowel loop separation • Cobblestone appearance to mucosa.

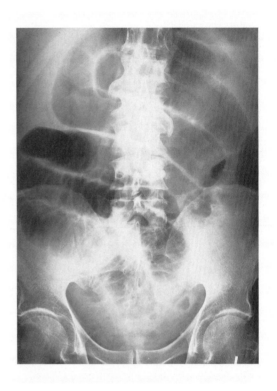

Fig. 21.15 Small bowel obstruction, supine AXR: Centrally located dilated small bowel loops • Multiple loops of small bowel • Greater than 3 cm but less than 5 cm in diameter • Valvulae conniventes (mucosal markings across full width of bowel) • Absence of gas within the large bowel (unless recent obstruction).

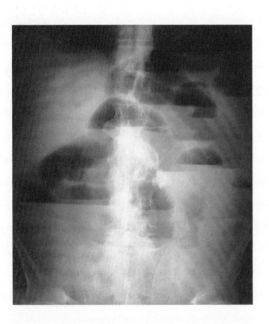

Fig. 21.16 Small bowel obstruction, erect AXR: Evidence of multiple distended small bowel loops containing air-fluid levels, sometimes referred to as a 'stepladder appearance'.

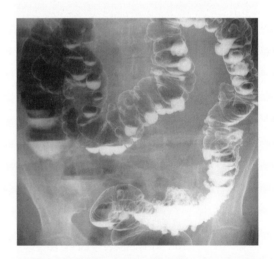

Fig. 21.17 Diverticular disease, barium enema: Smooth outpouchings of bowel (nearly always multiple and varying in size) with contrast within seen as a fluid level.

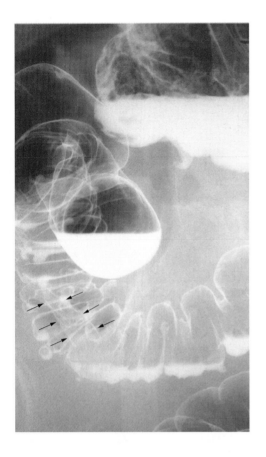

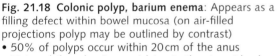

Fig. 21.18 Colonic polyp, barium enema: Appears as a filling defect within bowel mucosa (on air-filled projections polyp may be outlined by contrast) • 50% of polyps occur within 20 cm of the anus • Note subtle polyp (arrows) lying in the sigmoid colon, and coexistent diverticular disease • Associated diverticular disease can mask polyps as these are common coexisting pathologies.

Fig. 21.19 Familial adenomatous polyposis, barium enema: Bowel 'carpeted' with polyps, seen as small contrast filling defects • These polyps develop in the second decade of life.

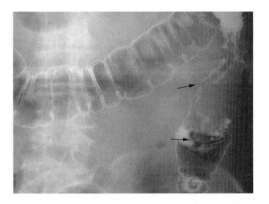

Fig. 21.20 Colorectal carcinoma, barium enema: Irregular strictured lesion distal to the splenic flexure • Proximal bowel dilation may herald impending intestinal obstruction • Classically an 'apple core' appearance with an annular carcinoma • Loss of normal bowel mucosa • Shouldering of the lesion.

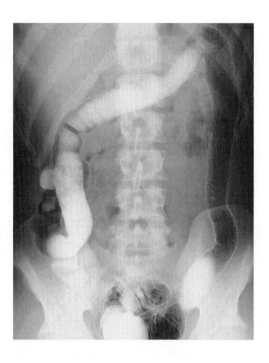

Fig. 21.21 Ulcerative colitis, barium enema: Confluent ulceration of the large bowel • Loss of haustral markings • Sometimes described as 'drain pipe' or 'lead pipe' colon.

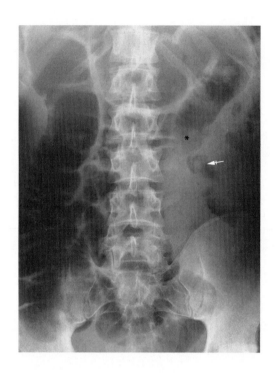

Fig. 21.22 Large bowel obstruction, supine AXR: The 'cut-off' between normal and obstructed colon is in the left colon (*) (see also Fig. 21.20) • Peripherally located dilated large bowel loops • Haustral markings (↔) • Few loops • Obstructed large bowel is greater than 5 cm in calibre (>9 cm for the caecum) • Cut-off point (indication of the level of the obstruction) • If the ileocaecal valve is incompetent gas may decompress into the small bowel • The cause of large bowel obstruction should be assumed to be colorectal cancer until proven otherwise.

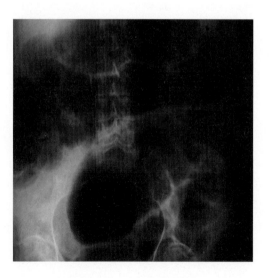

Fig. 21.23 Sigmoid volvulus, supine AXR: Characteristic 'coffee bean' sign—loops of dilated bowel twisted upon the bowel mesentery • Dilated proximal large bowel loops.

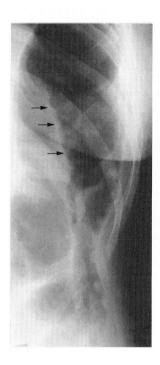

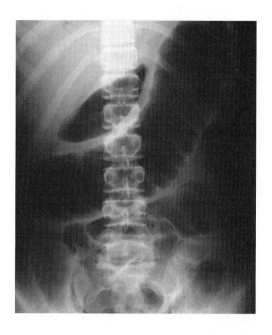

Fig. 21.24 Ischaemic colitis, supine AXR: Thumprinting due to oedema of the bowel mucosa (arrows) • Splenic flexure is the commonest location (due to site of arterial watershed) • Look for other evidence of cardiovascular disease on clinical examination.

Fig. 21.25 Toxic megacolon, thumbprinting on AXR: Dilated large bowel loops with preponderance for transverse colon • Thumbprinting of the bowel mucosa • Find this fast, as it is a cause of bowel perforation and with a high mortality.

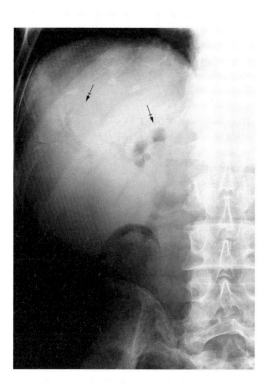

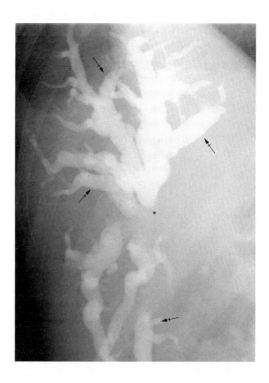

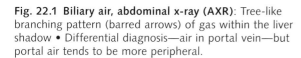

Fig. 22.1 Biliary air, abdominal x-ray (AXR): Tree-like branching pattern (barred arrows) of gas within the liver shadow • Differential diagnosis—air in portal vein—but portal air tends to be more peripheral.

Fig. 22.2 Cholangiocarcinoma, cholangiogram: Dilated intrahepatic biliary tree (barred arrows) • Widened biliary radicles • Look for filling defects within the biliary tree (*) • Look for continuity of the common bile duct and duodenum.

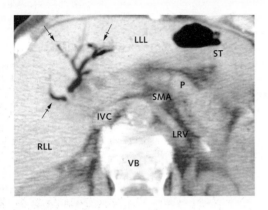

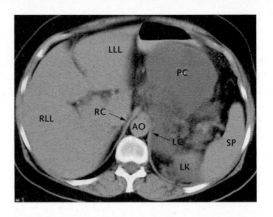

Fig. 22.3 Gas in biliary tree, CT abdomen: 'Tree-branching' pattern within the liver (barred arrows) • Look for absence of gallbladder or other biliary intervention • Look for biliary stent. (IVC, inferior vena cava; LLL, left lobe liver; LRV, left renal vein; P, pancreas; RLL, right lobe liver; SMA, superior mesenteric artery; ST, stomach; VB, vertebral body.)

Fig. 22.4 Pseudocyst of pancreas, CT abdomen: Typically located in the lesser sac between the stomach and pancreas (see Fig. 22.5). (AO, aorta; LC, left crus of diaphragm; LK, left kidney; LLL, left lobe liver; PC, pseudocyst; RC, right crus of diaphragm; RLL, right lobe liver; SP, spleen.)

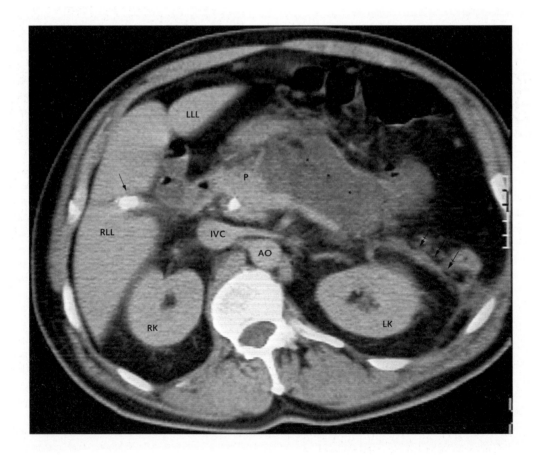

Fig. 22.5 Pancreatitis, CT abdomen: Normal pancreatic head/uncinate process (P) enhances normally • Necrotic and inflamed pancreatic body and tail are of lower attenuation (*) • Note inflamed left anterior pararenal plane (barred arrows) characteristic in pancreatitis • Gallstone (arrow) also seen within the gallbladder. (AO, aorta; IVC, inferior vena cava; LK, left kidney; LLL, left lobe liver; RK, right kidney; RLL, right lobe liver.)

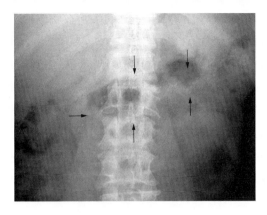

Fig. 22.6 Chronic pancreatitis, x-ray: Speckled calcification (arrows) traversing the upper abdomen • Location consistent with the head and body of the pancreas • Look for associated evidence of splenomegaly in portal hypertension.

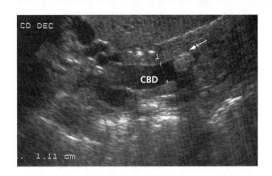

Fig. 22.8 Common bile duct (CBD), ultrasound: CBD—diameter approximately 6 mm (upper limit of normal) • If enlarged, look for evidence of intrahepatic duct dilatation or failure to taper normally at the lower end • Look for filling defects. (Barred arrow = calculus.)

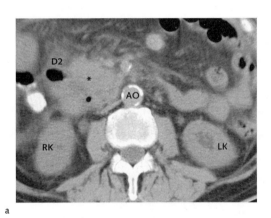

a

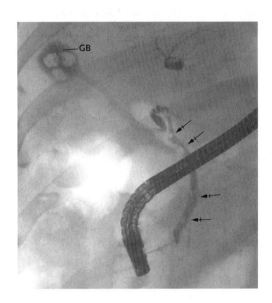

Fig. 22.9 Bile duct stones, ERCP: Multiple filling defects (gallstones, barred arrows) within the bile duct • Gallstones also in gallbladder (GB) • Postural imaging may be required to differentiate between calculus and air.

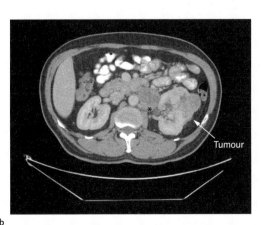

b

Fig. 22.7 (a) Carcinoma (*) of the head of pancreas, CT abdomen: Enlargement of pancreatic head (max. diameter 3 cm normally) • Evidence of distal enlargement of duct and gland atrophy • Absence of fat planes between mesenteric vessels and the pancreas • Metastatic disease, particularly liver, adenopathy. (AO, aorta; D2, second part of duodenum; LK, left kidney; RK, right kidney.) **(b)** Left renal carcinoma (←). Note left para-aortic lymphadenopathy (*).

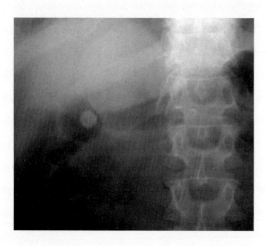

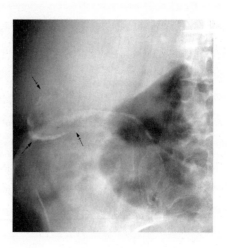

Fig. 22.10 Gallstones, AXR: Laminated calculus identified in the right upper quadrant • Approximately 10–20% gallstones are radiopaque and visible on abdominal radiograph.

Fig. 22.11 Porcelain gallbladder, AXR: Porcelain bladder calcification of wall of gallbladder • Association with malignancy 20% • Ultrasound may be indicated to exclude calculus.

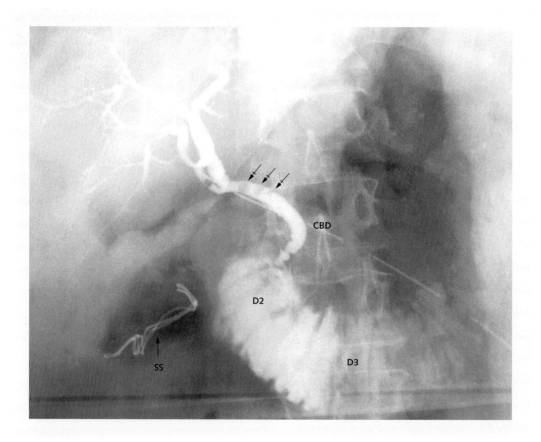

Fig. 22.12 Operative cholangiogram: Bile duct calculi (barred arrows) • Look for free flow into the duodenum. (CBD, common bile duct; D2, second part of duodenum; D3, third part of duodenum; SS, surgical swab.)

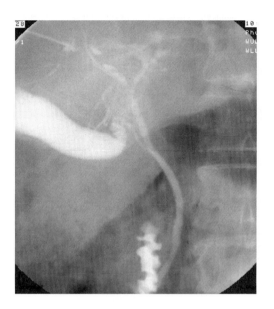

Fig. 22.13 Operative percutaneous transhepatic cholangiogram.

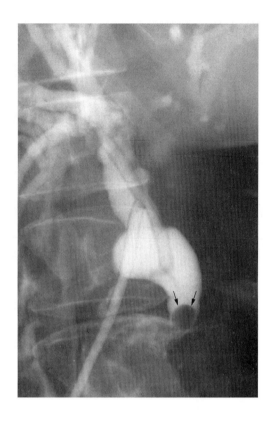

Fig. 22.14 Stone in bile duct (arrows), T-tube cholangiogram.

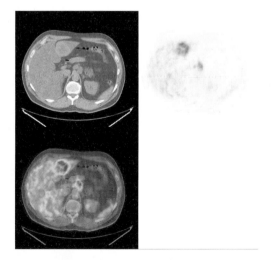

Fig. 22.15 Hepatic metastases, PET-CT scan (Courtesy of Dr J.C. Clarke): Top left: CT scan with metastases in the left lobe • Top right: PET scan showing FDG uptake in the lesion (arrows) • Bottom left: PET-CT fused image, showing the anatomical position of the metabolically active metastasis.

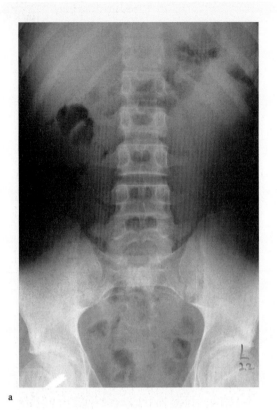
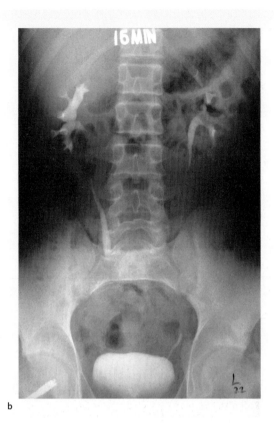

a

b

Fig. 22.16 **Normal intravenous urogram**: (a) Before contrast administration, ('control film') and (b) during examination, with kidneys and ureters visible.

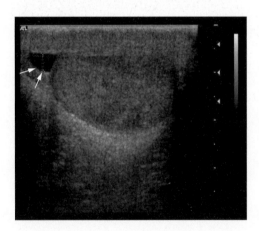

Fig. 22.17 **Ultrasound testes, epididymal cyst (arrows)**.

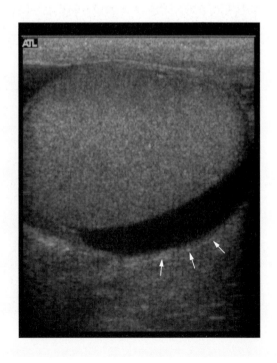

Fig. 22.18 **Ultrasound testes**: hydrocoele (arrows).

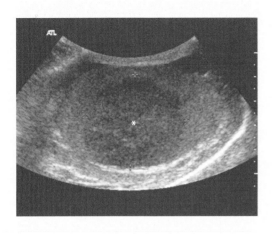

Fig. 22.19 Ultrasound testes: seminoma (*).

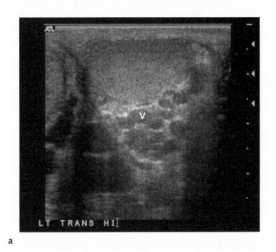

a

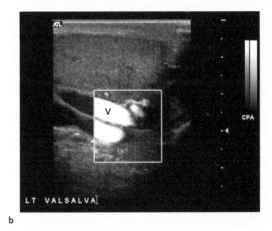

b

Fig. 22.20 Ultrasound testes: varicocoele (v). (a) Before, and (b) during Valsalva manoeuvre.

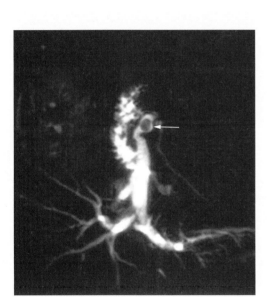

Fig. 22.21 MRI of stones in the bile duct (arrow).

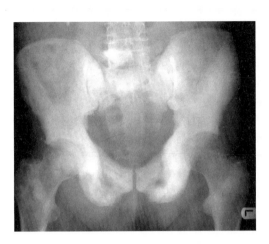

Fig. 23.1 Pelvic x-ray with sclerotic metastatic bone deposits: These may be bright (sclerotic) or dark (lucent) • Loss of trabecular pattern • Does not begin at a bone end (unlike Paget's disease) • Patient may have known history of primary tumour (in this case prostatic carcinoma).

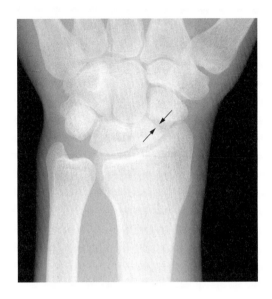

Fig. 23.2 Scaphoid fracture: Lucent line through waist of scaphoid (arrows) • Association: avascular necrosis of proximal fragment.

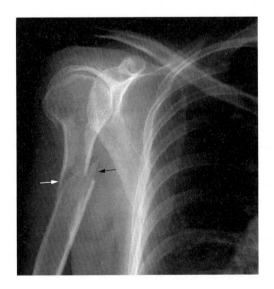

Fig. 23.3 Fracture of the shaft of the humerus: Loss of normal alignment • Fracture line visible (arrows) • Association with shaft fracture: radial nerve • Association with neck fracture: axillary nerve.

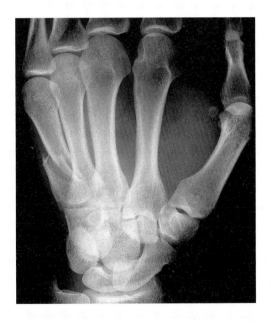

Fig. 23.4 Boxer's fracture, 5th metacarpal: Fracture line visible through 5th metacarpal bone.

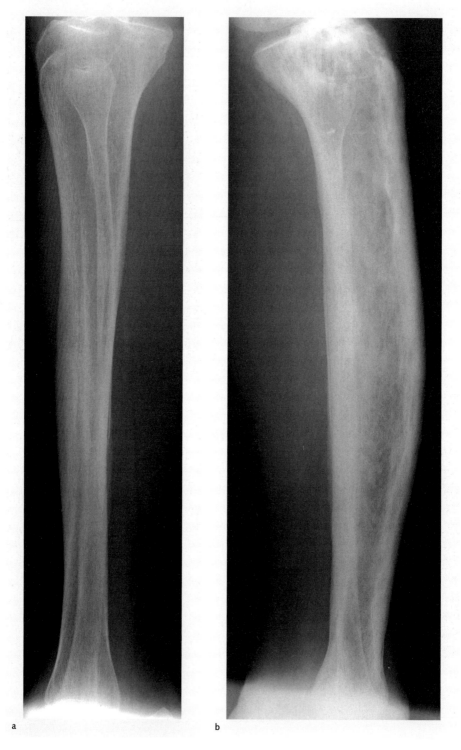

a   b

Fig. 23.5 (a) Normal tibia, (b) Paget's disease: Increased convexity of the tibia • Coarsening of the trabecular pattern • Association: sarcoma.

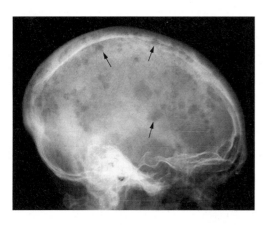

Fig. 23.6 Pepper-pot skull: Multiple lucencies present within the calvarium • Differential diagnosis: (1.) multiple myeloma (2.) hyperparathyroidism.

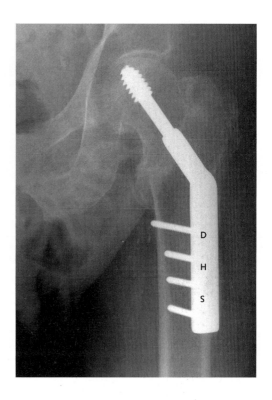

Fig. 23.7 Dynamic hip screw: Internal fixation device with screw through the femoral head and neck and secured to the femoral shaft with screws • Indication: extracapsular fracture with intact blood supply to femoral head.

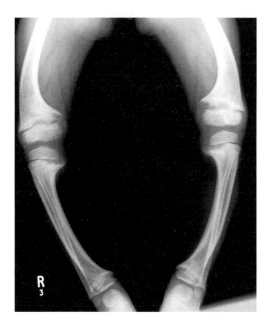

Fig. 23.8 Rickets: Convexity of both legs • Fraying, splaying and cupping at the epiphysis.

143

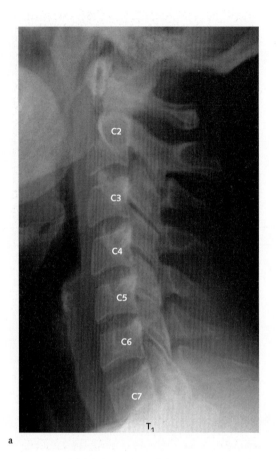

a

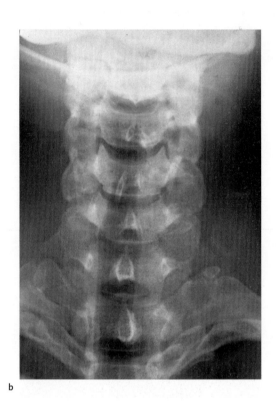

b

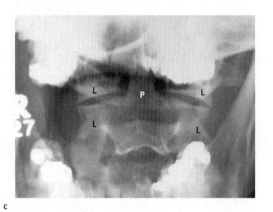

c

Fig. 23.9 Normal cervical spine x-rays: (a) Lateral; (b) anterior; (c) PEG views; P, odontoid peg • Confirm all 7 cervical vertebrae and T_1 are visible • Alignment of vertebrae maintained • Confirm on PEG view that the lateral masses of C_1 and C_2 (L) line up.

Fig. 23.10 Odontoid peg and teardrop fracture:
Aetiology is hyperextension • Both injuries unstable •
Other association of extension teardrop fracture is
hangman's fracture.

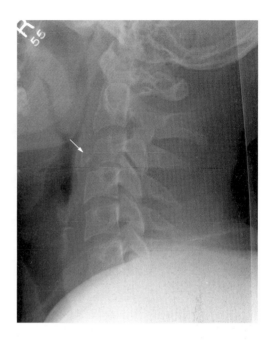

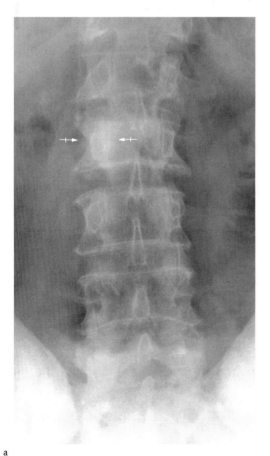

a

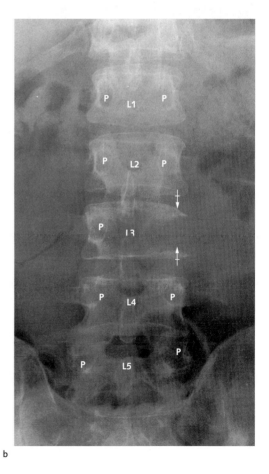

b

Fig. 23.11 (a) Osteoblastic L2 and (b) osteolytic L3 vertebrae metastases: Dense bone (arrows (a)) • Most likely
underlying cause is prostate or breast cancer or lymphoma • Osteolytic: lucent dark area in bone (arrows (b)) •
Absent left pedicle (P) at L3, classic appearance of an 'eye winking'.

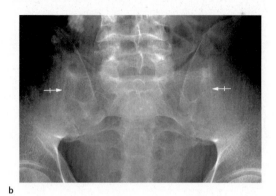

b

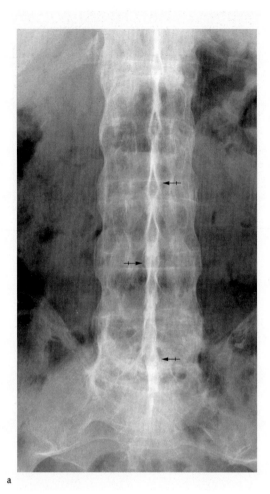

a

Fig. 23.12 Ankylosing spondylitis: (a) Bamboo spine with (b) sacroiliitis (arrows). Flowing syndesmophytes • Preservation of disc spaces • Multiple contiguous levels affected • Association: pseudofracture • Calcification of anterior spinous ligament (↔).

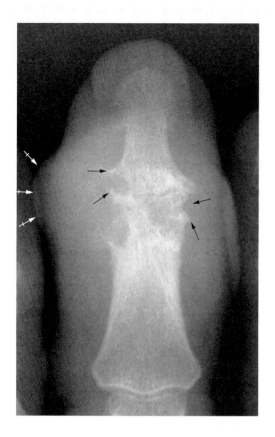

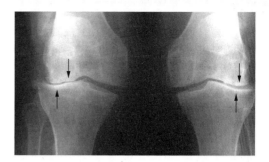

Fig. 23.15 Knees with osteoarthritis: Loss of joint space (arrows) • Osteophytic reaction • Sclerotic bone • Subchondral cysts.

Fig. 23.13 Gout: Asymmetric involvement of joints • Punched-out erosions away from the joint margin (→ arrows) • Soft tissue swelling (↔ arrows).

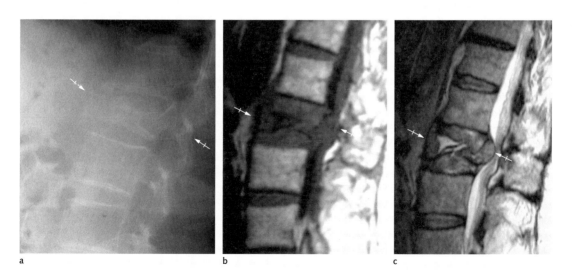

a   b   c

Fig. 23.14 Compression fracture of L2 (a) lateral spine x-ray, (b) T1, and (c) T2 weighted MRI scan: Loss of height in the vertebral body with wedging anteriorly • Decreased T1 and increased T2 signal • Posterior bulging against conus • Look for similar signal change at other levels • Clues to metastatic aetiology: normal bone density, other levels affected, known primary tumour, minimal trauma.

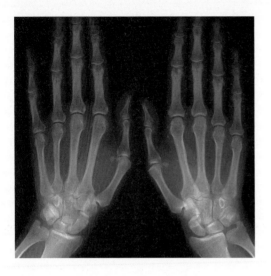

Fig. 23.16 Arachnodactyly in Marfan's syndrome: Elongated slender metacarpals • Metacarpal index greater than 8.4.

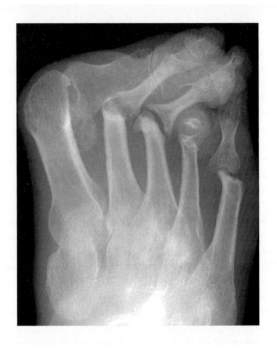

Fig. 23.17 Psoriatic arthropathy of the foot: Joint space narrowing with associated erosions centred at the MP and IP joint levels • History of psoriasis and overt skin changes.

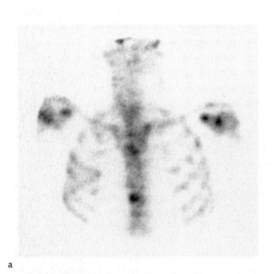

a

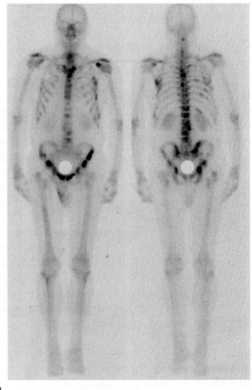

b

Fig. 23.18 Tc99m-MDP isotope bone scan demonstrating multiple metastases (a, b): Images acquired at 2–3 hours following injection • Multiple areas of increased isotope uptake • Asymmetrical distribution • History of known primary.

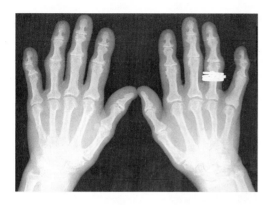

Fig. 23.19 X-ray of the hands in acromegaly: Hands enlarged • Metacarpals and phalanges spade shaped • Prominent tendinous insertions (entheses).

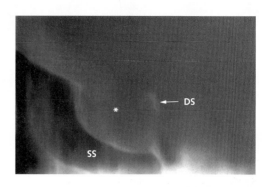

Fig. 23.20 Tomogram of enlarged pituitary fossa in acromegaly: Widening of the pituitary fossa (*) • Other features include erosion or destruction of the dorsum sella or posterior clinoids • Clinically: bitemporal hemianopia. SS: sphenoid sinus. DS: dorsum sellae.

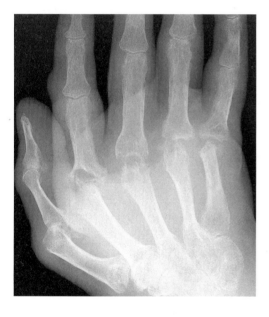

Fig. 23.21 X-ray of rheumatoid arthritis of the hand:
• Joint space narrowing centred on the MCP joints • Ulnar deviation, swan-necking, boutonnière deformity • Periarticular ostepenia • Bong erosions.

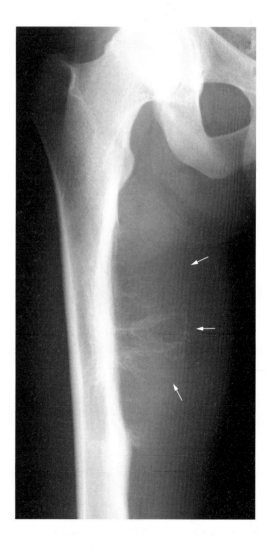

Fig. 23.22 X-ray of osteosarcoma of the femur (arrows): • Periosteal reaction • 'Godman's triangle' • 'Sunray spicules'.

149

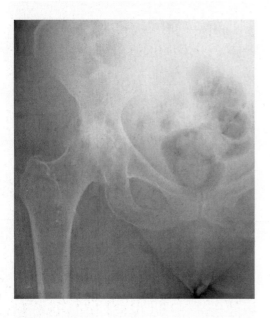

Fig. 23.23 X-ray of osteoarthritis of right hip: Loss of joint space on right side • Sclerotic reactive changes • Peripheral osteophytes • Subchondral cysts.

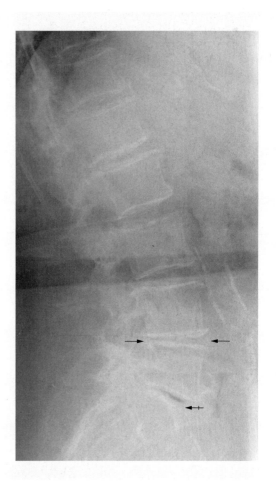

Fig. 23.24 Lateral x-ray—degenerative changes in lumbar spine: Disc space narrowing at the lower lumbar levels (→ arrows) • Osteophytic changes are present at the margins of the vertebral bodies • Gaseous degeneration of L5/S1 disc noted (↔ arrow) • Incidental aortic calcification noted.

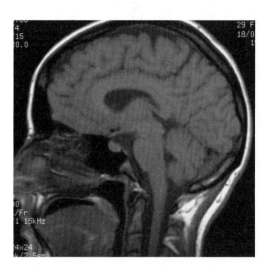

Fig. 24.1 Normal midline sagittal section, MRI scan (T1).

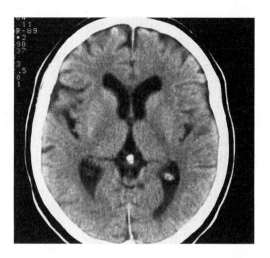

Fig. 24.2 Normal axial non-contrast CT scan at the level of the internal capsule.

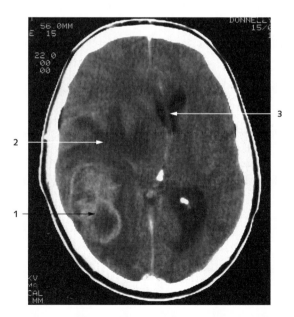

Fig. 24.3 Axial contrast enhanced CT brain glioma: High grade glioma (arrow 1) with surrounding low density oedema (arrow 2) • Heterogenous enhancement with central low density (necrosis) is typical of this tumour • Note marked mass effect with midline shift (arrow 3).

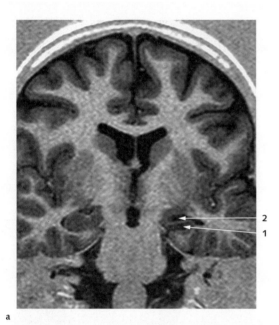

a

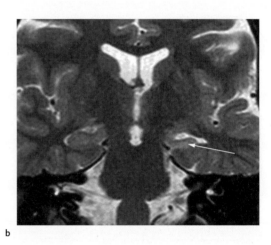

b

Fig. 24.4 Coronal MRI sequence through temporal lobes, (a) T1 inversion recovery and (b) T2 at the same level: Atrophic low signal hippocampus (a) (arrow 1) with prominent choroidal fissure (arrow 2)—typical features of mesial temporal sclerosis • Abnormal hippocampus high signal in (b) (arrow).

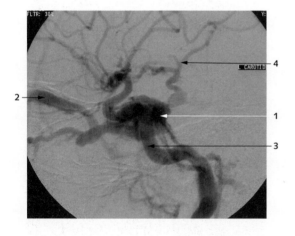

Fig. 24.5 Cerebral angiogram, lateral view, left common carotid artery caroticocavernous sinus fistula: Direct caroticocavernous sinus fistula • There is simultaneous filling of cavernous sinus (arrow 1), superior ophthalmic vein (arrow 2), and internal carotid artery (arrow 3) • Note cortical venous filling indicating high risk of brain haemorrhage without treatment (arrow 4).

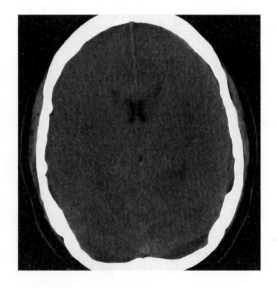

Fig. 24.6 Axial non-contrast CT brain: Lack of differentiation between grey and white matter structures, typical of global hypoxic ischaemic injury.

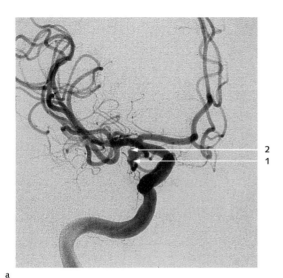

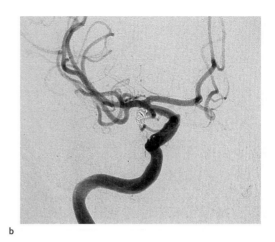

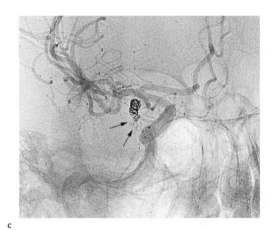

Fig. 24.7 Cerebral angiogram, intracerebral aneurysm (a) frontal view, right internal carotid artery, (b) aneurysm obliterated by coils (arrow), (c) same but unsubtracted image: Aneurysm in (a) arising at posterior communicating artery origin (arrow 1) • Note rupture bleb (arrow 2) • Coils in (b) and (c) clearly seen within the aneurysm (arrows).

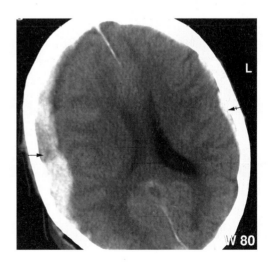

Fig. 24.8 Axial non-contrast CT brain: Large acute subdural haematoma (SDH) over right frontal and parietal lobes (arrow) • Crescentic shape is typical of SDH • Note smaller contralateral SDH (↔ arrow).

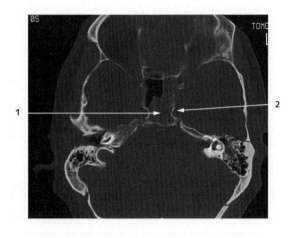

Fig. 24.9 Axial CT skull base fracture of sphenoid sinus (imaged on bone windows): Sphenoid sinuses opacified with blood (arrow 1) • Fracture in lateral wall left sphenoid sinus involving adjacent carotid canal (arrow 2).

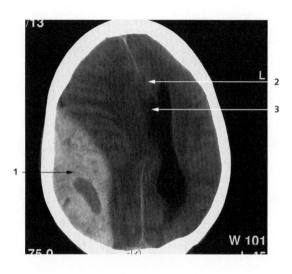

Fig. 24.11 Large acute extradural haematoma (arrow 1), axial CT: The biconvex shape is typical • Note marked mass effect with midline shift (arrow 2) and effacement of lateral ventricle (arrow 3).

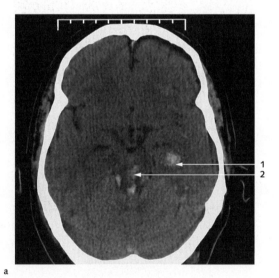

a

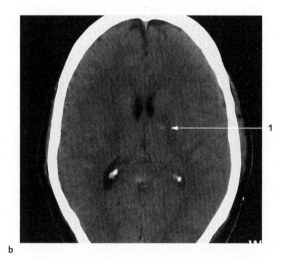

b

Fig. 24.10 Axial non-contrast CT brain: contusional haemorrhage and diffuse axonal injury (a) Contusional haemorrhage, medial left temporal lobe (arrow 1); brain stem haemorrhage involving midbrain (arrow 2). (b) Diffuse axonal injury; punctate haemorrhage at interface between left thalamus (grey matter) and internal capsule (white matter).

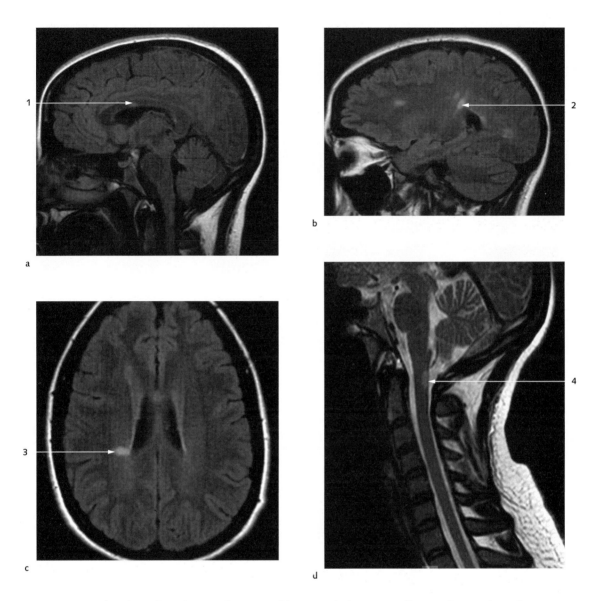

Fig. 24.12 Sagittal (a, b) and axial (c) T2 flair MRI of brain, and (d) T2 MRI of cervical spine demyelination:
Nodular foci typical of demyelination seen as bright areas in the corpus callosum (arrow 1 in (a)) and periventricular white matter (arrow 2 in (b) and 3 in (c)) • Demyelinating plaque posterior upper cervical cord (arrow 4 in (d)).

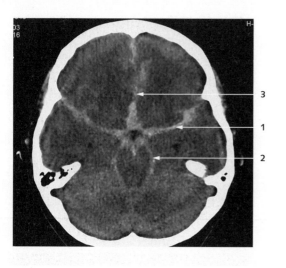

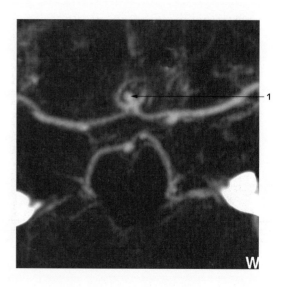

Fig. 24.13 Axial non-contrast CT brain with diffuse subarachnoid haemorrhage: Hyperdense acute haemorrhage in Sylvian fissures (arrow 1), basal cisterns (arrow 2) and interhemispheric fissure (arrow 3).

Fig. 24.14 CT angiogram: Aneurysm arising from anterior communicating artery (arrow 1).

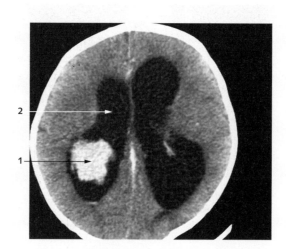

Fig. 24.15 Axial contrast enhanced CT brain: Choroid plexus papilloma within right lateral ventricle (arrow 1) • Note associated hydrocephalus (arrow 2).

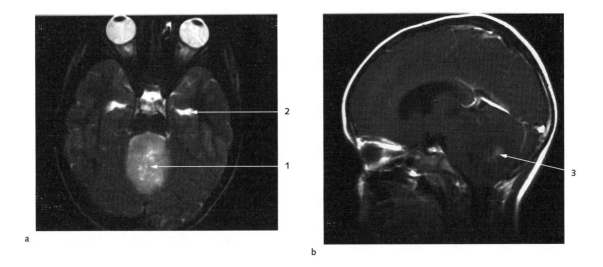

Fig. 24.16 Axial (a) and sagittal (b) T$_2$ weighted MRI of ependymoma in 4th ventricle: Bright on T2 MRI (arrow 1 in (a)) with patchy enhancement centrally (arrow 3 in (b)) • Note dilated temporal horns due to hydrocephalus (arrow 2 in (a)).

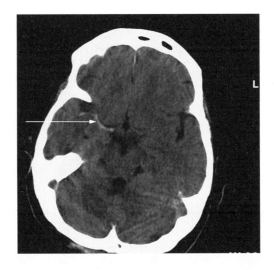

Fig. 24.17 Axial non-contrast CT brain cerebral thrombosis: Dense middle cerebral artery (arrow) due to acute thrombosis.

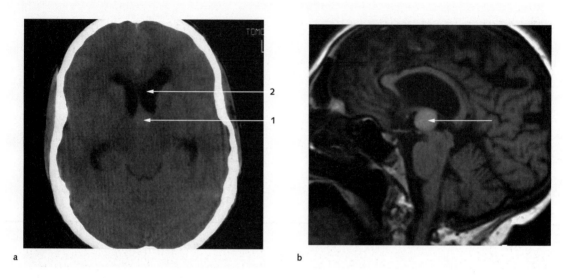

Fig. 24.18 (a) Axial non-contrast CT brain, (b) Non-contrast sagittal T1 MRI brain colloid cyst: (a) Hyperdense colloid cyst in base of septum pellucidum (arrow 1); note hydrocephalus (arrow 2). (b) Colloid cyst is seen as hyperintense (bright) mass (arrow).

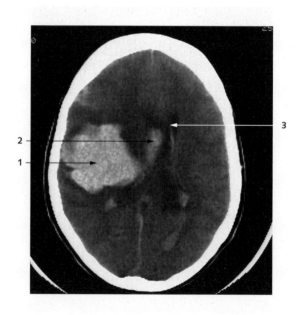

Fig. 24.19 Axial non-contrast CT brain intracranial haematoma. Large acute intracerebral haematoma (arrow 1) with intraventricular extension (arrow 2) and midline shift (arrow 3).

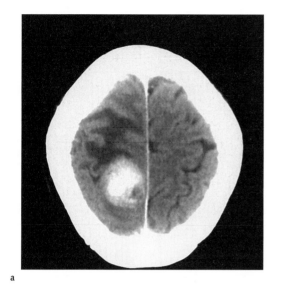

a

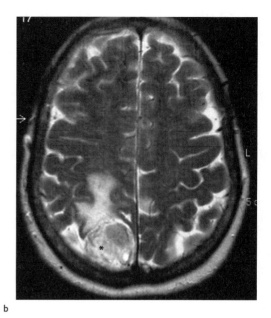

b

c

Fig. 24.20 Meningioma with adjacent oedema, (a) axial enhanced CT brain, (b) axial T2 and (c) contrast enhanced T1 MRI: Meningioma (*) better demonstrated on MRI, axial T2 (b) and contrast enhanced axial T1 (c) • Note characteristic enhancing dural tail in (arrow in c).

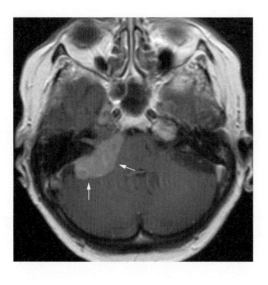

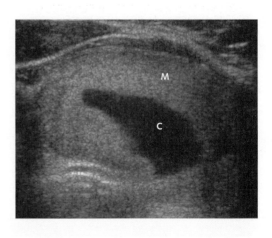

Fig. 24.22 Ultrasound scan: thyroid nodule. Solid mass (M) with a fluid centre (c).

Fig. 24.21 MRI scan: acoustic neuroma (arrows).

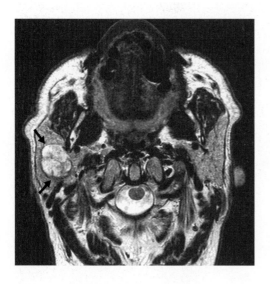

Fig. 24.23 Axial T$_2$ weighted MRI: pleomorphic adenoma • Well circumscribed mass in the right parotid gland (arrows).

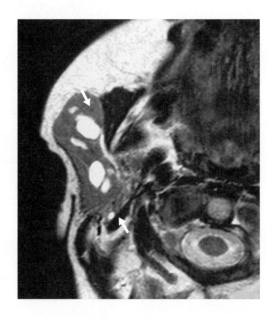

Fig. 24.24 Parotid gland MRI with Sjögren's syndrome. Axial T$_2$ weighted MRI: Sjögren's syndrome • Small cysts within the right parotid gland (arrows) • Association with Non-Hodgkins' lymphoma.

Fig. 24.25 Bilateral carotid body tumours on neck enhanced CT scan: Markedly enhancing masses (M) are noted bilaterally between the splayed internal carotid artery (ICA) and the external carotid artery (ECA).

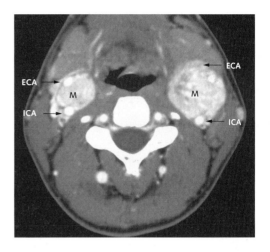

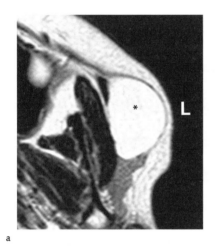

a

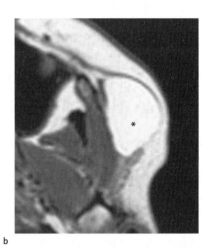

b

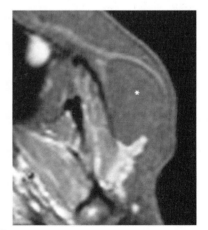

c

Fig. 24.26 MRI of a left cheek with lipoma, (a) axial T1 weighted, (b) axial T2 weighted, (c) axial fat suppressed: Lipoma (*) has normal characteristics of fat—high signal on T1 and T2 sequences and completely dark on fat suppression sequences.

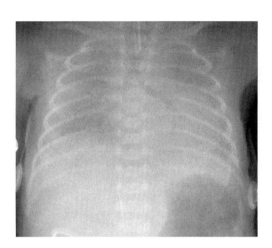

Fig. 25.1 Surfactant deficiency, CXR: Also known as respiratory distress syndrome or hyaline membrane disease • Affects premature infants less than 36 weeks gestational age • Non-compliant lungs are hypoinflated on the CXR • Collapsed alveoli combined with interstitial and alveolar oedema lead to bilateral lung opacities • Air bronchograms may be present • Can be complicated by pulmonary haemorrhage or air leaks.

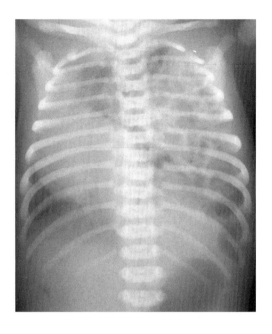

Fig. 25.2 Congenital diaphragmatic hernia, CXR: Most commonly Bochdalek hernias through the left, posterior pleuroperitoneal foramen • Usually diagnosed by antenatal sonography • Prognosis relates to the degree of pulmonary hypoplasia • Initially the CXR shows an opaque hemithorax due to fluid-filled loops of bowel which aerate with time • There is contralateral cardiomediastinal shift • The course of an orogastric tube will confirm if the stomach is lying in the thorax • **B**ochda**L**ek hernias lie at the **B**ack of the chest, are **B**ig, diagnosed in **B**abies and lie on the **L**eft side.

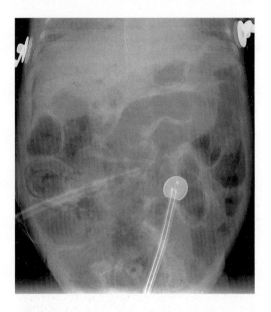

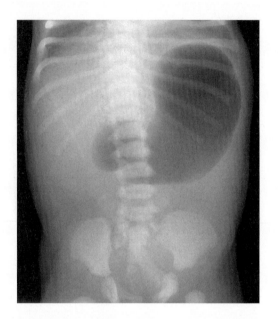

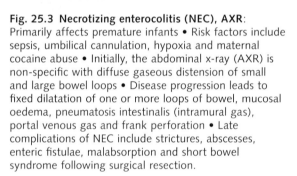

Fig. 25.3 Necrotizing enterocolitis (NEC), AXR:
Primarily affects premature infants • Risk factors include
sepsis, umbilical cannulation, hypoxia and maternal
cocaine abuse • Initially, the abdominal x-ray (AXR) is
non-specific with diffuse gaseous distension of small
and large bowel loops • Disease progression leads to
fixed dilatation of one or more loops of bowel, mucosal
oedema, pneumatosis intestinalis (intramural gas),
portal venous gas and frank perforation • Late
complications of NEC include strictures, abscesses,
enteric fistulae, malabsorption and short bowel
syndrome following surgical resection.

Fig. 25.4 Duodenal atresia, AXR: Shows the 'double
bubble' of the gas-filled stomach and duodenal cap •
80% are distal to the ampulla of Vater • One-third of
patients have Down's syndrome • May be diagnosed
antenatally • Maternal polyhydramnios and prematurity
are common • Neonatal duodenal obstruction may also
be due to a duodenal stenosis or web, annular pancreas
or small bowel malrotation and volvulus—all require
surgical management.

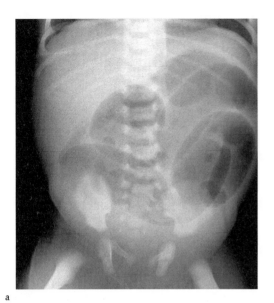

a

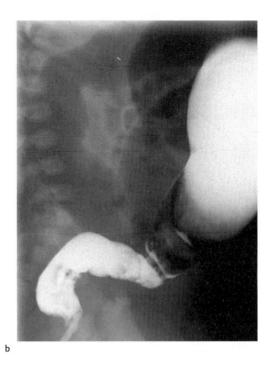

b

Fig. 25.5 (a) Low bowel obstruction, AXR; (b) Hirschsprung's disease, barium enema: Functional low bowel obstruction due to failure of caudad migration of neuroblasts in developing bowel • In 75% of cases the point of neuronal arrest is in the rectosigmoid colon • AXR shows low bowel obstruction, with multiple dilated loops of bowel down to the level of the obstruction, requires barium enema which may be diagnostic and therapeutic • Barium enema shows narrow aganglionic (distal) bowel with a funnel-shaped transition zone leading to dilated, normally innervated (more proximal) bowel • Irregular muscular contractions may be seen in the denervated rectum • In rectosigmoid Hirschsprung's disease, the sigmoid is more dilated than the rectum (reversal of the normal rectosigmoid ratio) • Complications of Hirschsprung's disease include bowel perforation and enterocolitis.

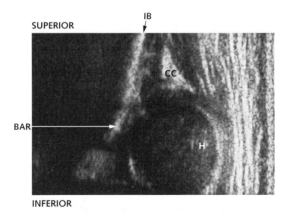

Fig. 25.6 Developmental dysplasia of the hip (DDH), ultrasound: Risk factors include breech delivery, positive family history of DDH, abnormal ligamentous laxity, maternal oligohydramnios and being a female infant • Ultrasound is the imaging method of choice up to 6 months of age • Coronal view with flexed hip shows the iliac bone as a straight vertical line (IB) • The lateral edge of the bony acetabular roof should be sharply angulated—it is rounded or flattened in dysplastic hips (as in this case) • The unossified femoral head (H) should be half to two-thirds covered by the acetabular roof • A dislocated femoral head is displaced superolaterally and posteriorly. (IB: innominate bone. BAR: bony acetabular roof. H: femoral head. CC: cartilage cap.)

165

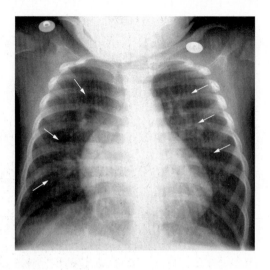

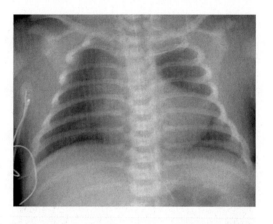

Fig. 25.8 Fallot's tetralogy: Four components to the tetralogy—a large VSD with an overriding, anteriorly displaced aorta, pulmonary outflow tract obstruction and consequent right ventricular hypertrophy • Right-sided aortic arch is seen in 25% of patients • CXR shows a 'boot-shaped' heart (coeur en sabot), the heart is moderately enlarged with an upturned apex • The main pulmonary artery segment is concave and the ascending aorta is dilated • The lungs are oligaemic due to right-to-left shunting of blood • Echocardiography, angiography and MRI are complementary imaging techniques that may be required.

Fig. 25.7 Atrioventricular septal defect (AVSD) (also referred to as an AV canal or endocardial cushion defect): Complete AVSD lesion has four components—ASD, VSD, cleft mitral valve and cleft tricuspid valve (leading to mitral and tricuspid regurgitation, respectively) • CXR shows cardiac enlargement, especially of the atria • Main pulmonary trunk is prominent and there is shunt vascularity • Pulmonary oedema may be superimposed • Shunt vascularity means both the pulmonary arteries (arrows) and veins are enlarged due to increase in volume of blood flowing through the pulmonary circulation • Shunt vascularity is synonymous with pulmonary plethora • Echocardiogram will confirm the diagnosis, angiography may also be required • Child with a left-to-right shunt is acyanotic—spotting this is key to formulating the differential diagnosis on CXR of patients with congenital heart disease • Other types of left-to-right shunt include ASD, VSD, PDA, AP window, PAPVD, coronary artery to right atrial fistula and anomalous origin of the left coronary artery when it arises from one the pulmonary arteries.

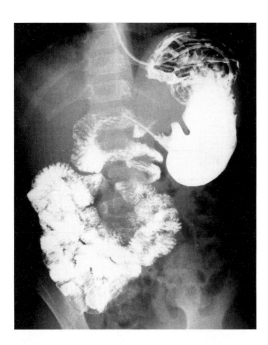

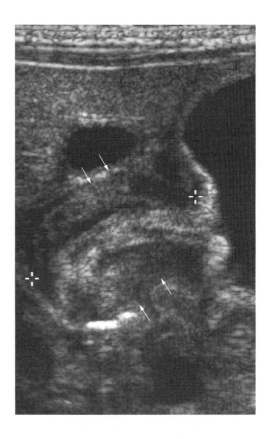

Fig. 25.9 Small bowel malrotation and volvulus, barium meal: Malrotation describes any variation in the position of the intestines and is associated with a short base to the small bowel mesentery which predisposes to midgut volvulus (twisting of the bowel and compromising its blood supply) • AXR findings are variable and non-diagnostic, upper GI contrast study is necessary to diagnose • The duodeno-jejunal flexure normally lies to the left of the left pedicles, at the same height as the duodenal cap, lying lower and to the right of midline in malrotation • Volvulus can totally occlude the bowel lumen and cause duodenal obstruction • Classically on an upper GI series, volvulus causes a 'corkscrew' pattern of the jejunum spiralling around the mesenteric vessels • Midgut volvulus is a life-threatening condition and requires emergency surgery after diagnosis.

Fig. 25.10 Hypertrophic pyloric stenosis, ultrasound: More common in first-born males who present between the ages of 4 and 6 weeks • Stomach should be filled with clear fluids before the ultrasound to act as an acoustic window through which to scan • Ultrasound features include a canal length >15 mm (white crosses) and a pyloric muscle thickness >2.5 mm (arrows) • Increased gastric peristalsis and failure of the pyloric canal to open may also be observed during real-time scanning • Barium meal examination occasionally required to confirm—shows elongated pyloric canal, with indentation of the gastric antrum and delayed gastric emptying.

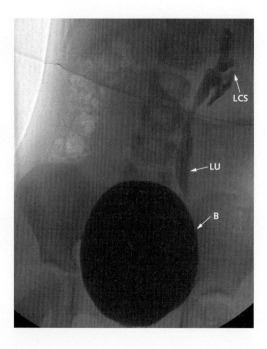

Fig. 25.11 Vesico-ureteric reflux (VUR), micturating cystourethrography (MCUG): May be detected using conventional MCUG, sonographic cystography, direct isotope cystography or indirect radionuclide cystography • VUR is graded I–V depending upon the severity, grade II+ reaches renal level • VUR is more common in the lower rather than the upper moiety of a duplex system • The bladder (B) and urethra are also demonstrated in a MCUG. (LCS, left (renal) collecting system; LU, left ureter.)

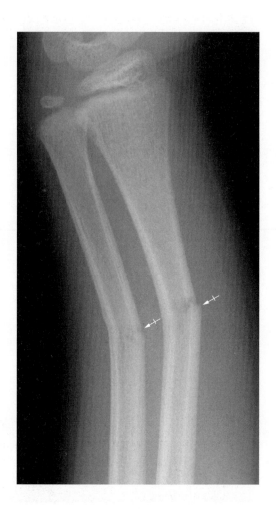

Fig. 25.12 Greenstick fracture of ulna and radius: Children's bones can tolerate more deformation than adult bones • Longitudinal compression of a bone results in plastic deformation and a bowing fracture • Continued force causes a torus (buckle) fracture, where the bone's cortex remains intact • Increasing the force further leads to a greenstick (incomplete) fracture in which there is a breach of the bone cortex on the convex side • Failure to remove the force will eventually lead to a complete fracture of the bone.

Fig. 25.13 Non-accidental injury (NAI): Skeletal trauma is most common in children <2 years of age • A skeletal survey *not* a 'babygram' is required • Isotope bone scans are useful if the history is suggestive of NAI and skeletal survey negative • CT defines associated intracranial and intra-abdominal injuries • Bone lesions which are of high specificity for NAI include metaphyseal ('corner' or 'bucket-handle') fractures, posterior rib fractures, scapular fractures, spinous process fractures and sternal fractures • All rib fractures are easier to see when they are healing (callus being visible) • Posterior fractures found just lateral to the costo-vertebral junction and usually associated with episodes of shaking • Bilateral subdural haematomas should be considered due to NAI until proven otherwise • Skeletal survey is required to look for other injuries.

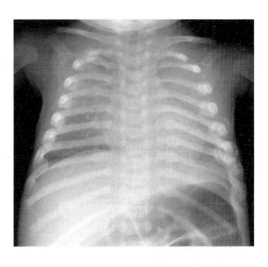

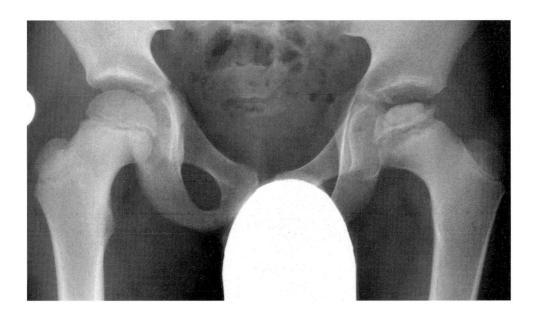

Fig. 25.14 Perthes' disease: Avascular necrosis of the capital femoral epiphysis, cause unknown • Is bilateral and asymmetric in 10% of cases • Early x-ray signs include fissure fractures, irregularity and increase in density of capital femoral epiphysis • Later x-ray changes include loss of height, fragmentation and sclerosis of the femoral head • Cysts may develop in the femoral neck, which broadens, and the outer portion of the dysplastic femoral head may not be covered by the acetabular roof • Reossification and remodelling of the femoral head occur with time, but deformity often persists • Further imaging with isotope bone scans and MRI is occasionally required to help make the diagnosis • Children with hip pathology may present with thigh or knee pain.

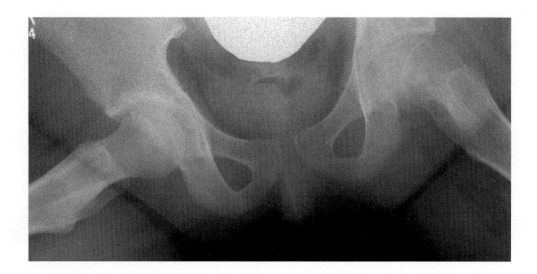

Fig. 25.15 Slipped upper femoral epiphysis (SUFE) (also known as SCFE—slipped capital femoral epiphysis): Represents a Salter Harris type I fracture through the proximal femoral growth plate • Both AP and 'frog-leg' lateral views of the hips are required for diagnosis • The AP view may show osteopenia of the femoral head and neck, widening of the growth plate and blurring of the metaphyseal margins • The frog-leg lateral shows the extent of posterior displacement of the femoral head • Avascular necrosis may complicate severe slips • Bilateral disease is not uncommon.

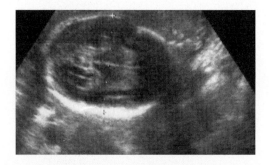

Fig. 25.16 Measurement of biparietal diameter during the second trimester, ultrasound: Transverse section of fetal skull, ultrasound calipers positioned from parietal bone to parietal bone.

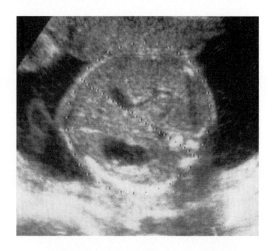

Fig. 25.17 Measurement of abdominal circumference, fetal ultrasound: Transverse section at the level of the stomach may be used in the third trimester to assess growth and estimate weight.

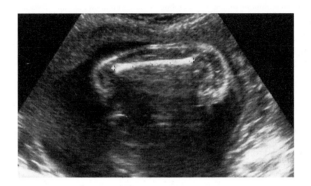

Fig. 25.18 Measurement of femur length, fetal ultrasound: Longitudinal view of femur obtained—measurement should correspond with biparietal diameter.

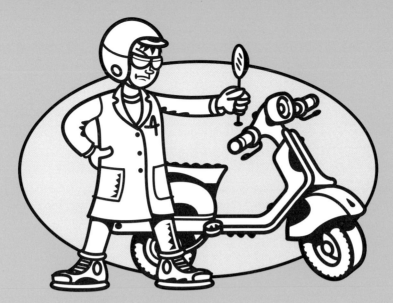

SELF-ASSESSMENT

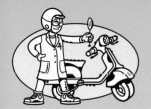

Multiple-choice Questions (MCQs)

Indicate whether each answer is true or false.

1. With regard to radiological contrast agents:

(a) Carbon dioxide is a recognized negative contrast agent
(b) Anaphylactic reactions occur in 1 in 20,000 patients
(c) Serum creatinine is routinely checked before IV contrast administration
(d) Iopamidol is routinely used as an IV contrast agent
(e) IV contrast should be avoided in those with penicillin allergy

2. Cryptogenic fibrosing alveolitis:

(a) Is best imaged by HRCT
(b) Has a reticulonodular appearance on CXR
(c) Predominantly affects the upper zones of the CXR
(d) Causes a 'shaggy' heart appearance on the CXR
(e) Is associated with chronic active hepatitis

3. Concerning bronchial carcinoma:

(a) CXR appearances are pathognomonic of carcinoma
(b) A cavitating lesion suggests squamous cell carcinoma
(c) CT imaging of the liver, adrenals and brain is routine
(d) Raised alkaline phosphatase is a recognized indication for a radioisotope bone scan
(e) Mediastinal lymph nodes of 2 cm on CT are significant

4. In rheumatoid arthritis:

(a) Loss of joint space typically occurs
(b) Bone cysts are commonly seen
(c) Periarticular osteoporosis occurs
(d) The DIP and PIP joints of the hand are characteristically affected
(e) A 'pencil in cup' deformity on a radiograph is typical

5. Following exposure to asbestos:

(a) A CXR is a useful screening tool
(b) Pleural plaques are seen in 50–80% of chest radiographs
(c) Reticulonodular appearance is a recognized feature
(d) Pleural effusions commonly occur
(e) Pleural thickening rarely occurs

6. With regard to jaundice:

(a) A diameter of 17 mm of the common hepatic duct on USS is within normal range
(b) MRCP reliably discriminates between calculus and carcinoma at the lower end of the CBD
(c) PTC may be used to image and take brushings of the biliary tree
(d) 80% of gallstones are visible on AXR
(e) ERCP is the gold standard for imaging the biliary tree

7. MRI:

(a) Is contraindicated in welders
(b) Can safely be undertaken in a patient with a hip prosthesis
(c) Makes use of the properties of helium ions in a magnetic field
(d) Of the brain has the equivalent radiation dose of 50 CXRs
(e) May be used as an alternative to contrast angiography in visualizing the carotid arteries

8. With regard to breast imaging:

(a) Microcalcification on mammography is pathognomonic of malignancy
(b) All women aged 45–65 are invited for screening
(c) Three radiographic projections are taken at screening
(d) Ultrasound is highly accurate in the diagnosis of fibrocystic disease
(e) A spiculated lesion on mammography is a characteristic finding of benign breast disease

9. In Crohn's disease:

(a) A labelled white cell scan assesses the extent of large bowel disease
(b) The ileocaecal segment is most commonly involved
(c) Small bowel enema gives a lower radiation dose than a small bowel series
(d) Bowel loop separation on small bowel series is a classical feature
(e) Sacroiliitis is a recognized feature

10. Regarding a thyroid mass:

(a) Ultrasound of the neck is essential
(b) A thoracic inlet view may help assess the extent of the lesion
(c) A solid nodule is usually malignant
(d) Metastases from a papillary carcinoma of the thyroid have a similar appearance on CXR to miliary TB
(e) FNAC is the investigation of choice

11. With regard to testicular lesions:

(a) Trans-scrotal ultrasound guided biopsy of the mass is useful
(b) Abdominal ultrasound is indicated in those with a left sided varicocoele
(c) CT abdomen and thorax is routinely used to stage malignant lesions
(d) Right sided varicocoeles are associated with renal cell carcinoma
(e) MRI abdomen is accurate in the localization of an undescended testicle

12. Radiological features of pulmonary embolus include:

(a) A vascular filling defect on CT pulmonary angiogram
(b) Pulmonary artery enlargement on CXR
(c) A matched defect on VQ scan
(d) Hyperexpansion of the contralateral lung on CXR
(e) The rare finding of Hampton's hump

13. In acute pancreatitis:

(a) A sentinel loop on AXR is usually seen
(b) A pseudocyst is best seen on plain radiograph
(c) CT with contrast enhancement is necessary to exclude pancreatic necrosis
(d) A small pneumoperitoneum is an associated feature
(e) Ultrasound is reliable in evaluating the degree of pancreatic oedema

14. The following are true with respect to the silhouette sign on the CXR:

(a) Right upper lobe consolidation typically obscures the right heart border
(b) Lingular consolidation manifests as loss of the left heart border
(c) Left lower lobe collapse causes loss of the left heart border
(d) Right middle lobe consolidation obscures the right hemidiaphragm
(e) Left upper lobe collapse obscures the aortic knuckle

15. Breast masses:

(a) Are best imaged by mammography in women over 35 years old
(b) Are identified on mammography if over 10 mm in more than 90% of cases
(c) Are biopsied by stereotactic guidance if hard to palpate clinically
(d) Are clearly seen on ultrasound when cystic in nature
(e) Are investigated by triple therapy of imaging, biopsy and FNAC

16. Features of osteoarthritis of the hip seen on x-ray include:

(a) Narrowing of the joint space
(b) Periarticular erosions
(c) Subchondral bone cysts
(d) Periarticular osteopenia
(e) Osteoclast formation

17. In osteoporosis:

(a) There is irreversible loss of bone architecture
(b) The degree of osteopenia can be predicted from the plain radiograph
(c) A DEXA scan T-score of greater than −2.5 equals osteoporosis
(d) Vertebral wedge compression fractures are often seen at the lumbar spine
(e) MRI can reliably distinguish new from old fractures

18. The following are true of bony metastases:

(a) Sclerotic metastases are more common than lytic
(b) Sclerotic metastases most commonly arise from the testis
(c) They are the commonest cause of pathological fractures
(d) Lytic metastases are seen as areas of radio-opacity on plain x-ray
(e) They may be confused with the lesions of multiple myeloma on plain radiograph

19. Nephrocalcinosis is seen in the following conditions:

(a) Medullary sponge kidney
(b) Polycystic kidney disease
(c) Hypoparathyroidism
(d) Renal tubular acidosis
(e) Sarcoidosis

20. The following may give rise to calcification on CXR:

(a) Varicella pneumonia
(b) Tuberculosis
(c) Hyperthyroidism
(d) Hypercalcaemia
(e) Sarcoidosis

21. **The following matching statements are correct with regard to radiation dose equivalents:**

(a) 1 CXR = a return flight from London to Paris
(b) 1 AXR = 25 CXRs
(c) CT scan of chest = 1 year of background radiation
(d) Barium enema = 200 CXRs
(e) CT of abdomen = 500 CXRs

22. **With regard to gastrointestinal volvulus:**

(a) Gastric volvulus is the most common site
(b) A caecal volvulus commonly leads to faecal peritonitis
(c) A sigmoid volvulus gives rise to the 'coffee bean' sign on AXR
(d) Barium enema is a suitable investigation
(e) Intussusception is a recognized association

23. **In cardiac failure:**

(a) CXR signs arise due to an increase in pulmonary wedge pressure
(b) Kerley A and B lines may be seen
(c) Lower lobe diversion is a recognized feature
(d) The degree of cardiomegaly on CXR reflects ejection fraction
(e) TOE is superior to TTE for assessment of left ventricular function

24. **Regarding CT imaging:**

(a) Following a CT of the abdomen the risk of acquiring cancer increases to 1 in 2000
(b) HRCT uses a slice thickness of 1 mm compared with 10 mm slices on conventional pulmonary CT
(c) Helical CT allows multiplanar reconstruction
(d) HRCT is rarely of use in interstitial lung disease
(e) CT is contraindicated in patients with pacemaker devices

25. **Concerning peripheral vascular disease:**

(a) A 10 cm long aorto-iliac stenosis is suitable for stenting
(b) Angioplasty is superior to bypass surgery for distal disease
(c) An iodine-based contrast agent is used in 25–50% of patients undergoing angiography
(d) An ABPI of 0.5–0.8 is associated with claudication
(e) Angioplasty has a limb loss rate of 10%

26. **Biliary gas on AXR.**

(a) Is seen in acute cholangitis
(b) Is a recognized association in acute pancreatitis
(c) Is a routine imaging finding following ERCP and sphincterotomy
(d) Is a recognized radiographic feature of gallstone ileus
(e) Is seen in necrotizing enterocolitis

27. **Regarding imaging of gallstone disease:**

(a) USS abdomen is the investigation of choice
(b) Approximately half of gallstones are seen on AXR
(c) Gallstones are seen as filling defects on CT of the abdomen
(d) An acoustic shadow is a characteristic finding on ultrasound
(e) A wall echo shadow implies chronic cholecystitis

28. **Potential causes of a cavitating lesion on CXR are:**

(a) Squamous cell bronchial carcinoma
(b) Pulmonary contusion
(c) Empyema
(d) Tuberculosis
(e) Lung abscess

29. **Pneumothorax:**

(a) May be allowed to resolve spontaneously
(b) Is seen best on the inspiratory chest film
(c) Always requires a daily CXR initially
(d) If under tension produces diaphragmatic elevation
(e) Is a recognized complication of nephrectomy

30. **On the normal supine AXR:**

(a) The kidneys lie between the L1 and L4 vertebrae
(b) A gastric pseudotumour is a normal finding
(c) Large bowel diameter is less than 5 cm
(d) Gas can be observed within the biliary tree
(e) The outline of the abdominal aorta is usually visible

31. **On the normal posteroanterior CXR:**

(a) The left hemidiaphragm is lower than the right
(b) Loss of the right heart border indicates right lower lobe consolidation
(c) The left hilum is higher than the right
(d) Ten anterior ribs should be visible in the mid-clavicular line
(e) The mediastinum to thorax ratio is less than 25%

32. **The level of the diaphragm may be elevated in:**

(a) Hepatosplenomegaly
(b) Bronchial carcinoma
(c) Following treatment for tuberculosis
(d) Apical lung fibrosis
(e) Subphrenic abscess

33. Recognized features of mitral stenosis on CXR include:

(a) Cardiomegaly
(b) Splaying of the subcarinal angle
(c) A double right heart border
(d) Prominence of the right atrial appendage
(e) An enlarged aortic knuckle

34. CXR signs of tuberculosis include:

(a) Fibrosis predominantly in the lower zones
(b) Pericardial effusion
(c) Miliary shadowing
(d) Pleural calcification
(e) Overinflated lungs

35. A complete 'white out' of the lung on CXR:

(a) May follow treatment for bronchial carcinoma
(b) Could be due to a haemopneumothorax
(c) Can occur in severe fibrosing alveolitis
(d) Is a recognized feature of ARDS
(e) May be due to advanced mesothelioma

36. A mediastinal mass on CXR:

(a) If in the middle mediastinum can obliterate the paratracheal stripe
(b) Commonly causes tracheal shift
(c) May cause superior vena cava obstruction
(d) Is a recognized feature in a patient with ptosis
(e) Occasionally leads to Ortner's (cardiovocal) syndrome

37. Bilateral hilar lymphadenopathy:

(a) Is seen in less than 30% of cases of sarcoidosis
(b) May follow pulmonary hypertension
(c) Is usually symmetrical in TB
(d) Is found in association with paratracheal nodes in sarcoidosis
(e) Is a feature of ARDS pneumonia

38. Imaging abdominal aortic aneurysms:

(a) Is routinely undertaken in smokers over the age of 60 years
(b) Is undertaken annually in those with a known 5 cm aneurysm
(c) By contrast enhanced CT is advisable preoperatively
(d) Shows 80% to be infrarenal
(e) May be first noted incidentally on AXR

39. Concerning carotid artery imaging:

(a) It is recommended in all patients suffering a TIA
(b) Carotid angiography is the gold standard imaging modality
(c) Those found to have a 70% stenosis and are asymptomatic should have surgery
(d) It should only be undertaken if the patient is a surgical candidate
(e) It may be used to diagnose a carotid body tumour

40. With respect to coarctation of the aorta:

(a) Rib notching is a classical feature
(b) Aortic dilatation is seen distal to the coarctation
(c) It is usually associated with cardiac failure
(d) Classically occurs at the level of the brachiocephalic artery
(e) Peripheral pruning of the lungs is a recognized feature

41. Concerning interstitial lung disease:

(a) Tenting of the diaphragms is seen in lower zone fibrosis
(b) Cryptogenic organizing pneumonitis involves the lung periphery
(c) Bleomycin causes upper zone fibrosis
(d) Alveolar proteinosis is seen centrally on CXR
(e) Sarcoidosis may progress to honeycomb lung

42. The aortic knuckle:

(a) If right sided is a recognized normal variant
(b) Is not seen clearly in left upper lobe consolidation
(c) Is prominent with atrial septal defect
(d) Is less prominent in tetralogy of Fallot
(e) Has a classical 'double hump' in patent ductus arteriosus (PDA)

43. Regarding imaging of children with urinary tract infection:

(a) Proteus infections are associated with the formation of renal tract calculi
(b) A renal pelvis diameter of >2 cm is considered significant for hydronephrosis on renal tract ultrasound
(c) One of the methods for performing a nuclear cystogram involves the direct injection of 99m-pertechnetate into the bladder
(d) Over 90% of children with a documented UTI will have VUR
(e) CT scans are routinely used in the evaluation of children with documented UTIs

44. Regarding neonates:

(a) All infants should pass meconium within 24 hours of birth
(b) The commonest site for the transition zone in Hirschsprung's disease is at the splenic flexure
(c) 75% of children with cystic fibrosis present as neonates with meconium ileus
(d) Meconium peritonitis is a complication of meconium ileus
(e) The 'double bubble' appearance is seen on plain AXR in infants with ileal atresia

45. The limping child:

(a) The incidence of DDH is increased in children born with talipes
(b) The femoral head ossifies at around the time of a child's first birthday
(c) Transient synovitis is usually due to a *Staphylococcus aureus* infection involving the hip joint
(d) An isotope bone scan can show a reduced uptake of tracer in the femoral head in children with septic arthritis
(e) Discitis is most commonly due to infection with *S. aureus*

46. Consider the following statements concerning slipped capital femoral epiphysis (SCFE)

(a) SCFE is best demonstrated on the 'frog-leg' lateral view
(b) The femoral head slips anteriorly in SCFE
(c) Renal osteodystrophy is a risk factor for SCFE
(d) Avascular necrosis (AVN) of the femoral head is a complication of SCFE
(e) SCFE is bilateral in 50% of cases

47. In neonates:

(a) In surfactant deficiency there is lung hypoinflation
(b) Congenital diaphragmatic hernias are more common on the left side
(c) Duodenal atresia is usually proximal to the ampulla of Vater
(d) Maternal polyhydramnios is a risk factor for the development of DDH
(e) Infants with isolated left-to-right shunts are cyanosed

48. Consider the following statements regarding acute neurological deficit:

(a) In the absence of haemorrhage, CT is often normal within 3 hours of onset
(b) Intracerebral haemorrhage is best seen following IV contrast
(c) Basal ganglia haemorrhage is usually due to hypertension
(d) Anterior cerebral artery aneurysms rupture into the sylvian fissure
(e) Paraparesis is a common presenting complaint

49. With regard to head trauma:

(a) MRI is the investigation of choice
(b) A Glasgow Coma Scale of 13 is an indication for CT
(c) Extradural haematoma results from trauma to the middle meningeal artery
(d) Venous extradural haematomas are usually in the posterior fossa
(e) Extradural haematoma is classically 'lens' shaped on CT

50. Regarding headache:

(a) Hypodensities in the subarachnoid spaces are classical findings of subarachnoid haemorrhage on unenhanced CT
(b) The commonest cause of subarachnoid haemorrhage is an AVM
(c) Colloid cyst typically obstructs the aqueduct of Sylvius
(d) The commonest location for paediatric CNS malignancy is supratentorial
(e) Headache, maximal in the evening, is suspicious of underlying malignancy

179

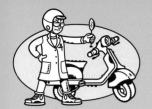

1. Write short notes on AXR calcification.

2. Outline how to approach the assessment and presentation of a CXR in an exam setting.

3. Explain the role of imaging in the assessment and preoperative management of an abdominal aortic aneurysm (AAA) patient.

4. Outline your algorithm for the imaging investigations of a jaundiced patient.

5. Draw up a chart comparing the radiological features of small and large bowel obstruction on AXR.

6. A 3 cm mass is noted on the chest X-ray (CXR) of a 53-year-old female smoker. What further imaging would you request?

7. Write short notes on the role of the radiologist in the investigation and treatment of lower limb peripheral vascular disease.

8. Outline the work-up of a female patient with a breast lump with emphasis on the role of imaging.

9. The consultant on your ward asks you to talk to the medical students about the silhouette sign on CXR. Make notes.

10. What would you expect to see on a CXR of a mitral stenosis patient? Explain why these features occur.

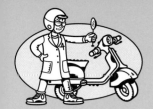

1. Theme: Altered bowel habit

(a) Ulcerative colitis
(b) Crohn's disease
(c) Colorectal carcinoma
(d) Irritable bowel syndrome
(e) Large bowel obstruction
(f) Gastroenteritis
(g) Diverticulitis
(h) Scleroderma
(i) Ischaemic colitis

Instruction: *For each scenario described below, choose the SINGLE most likely diagnosis from the above list of options. Each option may be used once, more than once, or not at all.*

1. A 65-year-old retired policeman consults his GP with a 3-month history of diarrhoea associated with bloating sensations. His weight and appetite are stable. He admits to a variable diet over the years. He has been stressed lately following the death of his wife. O/E: Unremarkable. PR: normal. Proctoscopy: normal. Hb 9.6 g/dL, WCC 13.5 × 10⁹/L, CEA 3.4 ng/mL. ☐

2. A 23-year-old university student attends the University Health Service with altered bowel habit in the run up to her final examinations. Her weight and appetite are stable, but she admits to intermittent crampy abdominal pains. Her periods are regular. O/E: Unremarkable. CRP, WCC and alpha-1-glycoprotein are normal. Barium enema was normal at outpatients. ☐

3. A 26-year-old accountant attends surgical outpatients complaining of ongoing diarrhoea with the occasional bloody stool. He has weight loss of 6 kg and a reduced appetite over the past 2 months. He is currently on ibuprofen for joint pains, but is otherwise well. In the past 3 months he has taken 9 days of sick leave. O/E: His lips are swollen. The LIF is mildly tender. No masses palpable. Proctoscopy: normal. Alpha-1-glycoprotein 3.6 kU/L. He is currently awaiting a barium enema and small bowel series. ☐

4. A 45-year-old postman attends outpatients with a 3-month history of altered bowel habit, reduced appetite and occasional PR bleeding. He drinks 38 units of alcohol a week. His younger brother in Australia attends the hospital for a 'bowel problem'. O/E: Tender LIF with a fullness in the same area. 2 cm hepar. Flexible sigmoidoscopy reveals an erythematous rectosigmoid. Barium enema: no focal lesion seen. ☐

5. A 59-year-old man is admitted from the clinic with a 2-month history of tenesmus and a 4 kg weight loss over the past month. Admission bloods Hb 9.6 g/dL, WCC 9.1 × 10⁹/L, MCV 69.2 fL, K 3.2 mmol/L, Na 137 mmol/L, urea 6.0 mmol/L, creatinine 79 Mmol/L. O/E PR: tender, blood on glove, and impacted stool (poor cooperation from patient). CEA 7.6 ng/mL. Barium enema: 'apple core stricture'. ☐

2. Theme: Jaundice

(a) Cholangiocarcinoma
(b) Hepatic metastases
(c) Hepatocellular carcinoma
(d) Pancreatic carcinoma
(e) Gallbladder carcinoma
(f) Biliary colic
(g) Alcoholic hepatitis
(h) Hepatic cirrhosis
(i) Chronic pancreatitis
(j) Liver abscess

Instruction: *For each scenario described below, choose the SINGLE most likely diagnosis from the above list of options. Each option may be used once, more than once, or not at all.*

1. A 64-year-old former miner is admitted with painless jaundice and a distended abdomen. He admits to 10 kg weight loss over the past 2 months. His admission LFTs showed an obstructive picture. CA 19-9: 686 U/mL. He drinks 20 units of alcohol per week and is an ex-smoker of 3 years. ☐

2. A 56-year-old lady is admitted with jaundice, but is otherwise well. She has a history of hepatitis C acquired whilst a missionary in Africa 30 years ago. O/E: 2 cm firm hepar. No ascites or splenomegaly. USS: multiple focal lesions within the liver, confirmed on CT. ☐

3. A 48-year-old salesman is admitted with severe epigastric pain of 2 days' duration. He admits to smoking 30 cigarettes a day and being a 'moderate drinker'. He is not aware of any change in the colour of his stools or urine. He has no past medical history and claims to have never been in hospital before. O/E: Mildly icteric with central abdominal discomfort. His amylase is 560 U/L. Your colleague informs you that she had problems controlling this patient's analgesic demands overnight. AXR: spiculated calcification on the left side extending over the midline. ☐

4. A 71-year-old woman is transferred from a peripheral hospital following a 10-day admission with jaundice. An ERCP was performed which demonstrated mild extrahepatic duct dilatation. Her LFTs were of a mixed picture. You note that previous imaging investigations were performed 7 years ago whilst an inpatient in your hospital. An old AXR report commented: 'No obstruction or extraluminal gas. Porcelain gallbladder'. ☐

5. A 49-year-old woman is admitted on the acute surgical 'take-in' with a 3-day history of jaundice, fever and lethargy. O/E: Overweight, icteric with RUQ tenderness. No abdominal masses are palpable. Her chart shows a pyrexia of above 38°C with temperature spikes. She admits to avoiding fatty foods since her last admission 4 months ago when she underwent 'tests'. Old notes reveal these to be USS abdomen and ERCP. WCC 18.7×10^9/L, CRP 109 mg/L. ☐

3. **Theme: Chest pain**

(a) Myocardial infarct
(b) Pulmonary embolus
(c) Pericarditis
(d) Left lower lobe pneumonia
(e) Rib fracture
(f) Oesophageal reflux disease
(g) Aortic dissection
(h) Costochondritis
(i) Angina pectoris
(j) Herpes zoster

Instruction: *For each scenario described below, choose the SINGLE most likely diagnosis from the above list of options. Each option may be used once, more than once, or not at all.*

1. A 48-year-old housewife is admitted with left-sided chest discomfort, sharp in nature, which is worse on coughing. She has no sputum. She takes the oral contraceptive pill and propranolol hydrochloride (Half-Inderal LA). Her father and uncle died in their sixties from 'heart attacks'. She smokes 30 cigarettes a day. ECG: sinus tachycardia and RBBB. D-dimer 0.71 mg/L, troponin I 0.01 mg/L. CXR: NAD. ☐

2. A 58-year-old insulin-dependent diabetic is admitted at the request of his GP. He has been complaining of intermittent central chest pain for the past month. He is a poor historian but claims he hasn't noticed any relationship to the pain. He has suffered from AF and hypertension for 6 years. He currently takes digoxin, atenolol, diclofenac and simvastatin. O/E: BMI 31, no chest wall tenderness, HS I + II + ESM in aortic area. No clinical evidence of DVT. HbA$_{1c}$ 10.5%, random glucose 13.2 mmol/L, digoxin level 1.3 mmol/L. ECG:1 mm depression in leads V1–V6. CXR: NAD. ☐

3. A 45-year-old Moroccan man (working in the local chicken factory) attended A&E with central chest discomfort. His English is broken, but you establish this has been a problem for the past week and that it is sharp in nature—'like a knife, doctor'. He has no recent trauma. Examination is unremarkable. CXR: scarring of right apex and calcified hilar nodes. You return to the patient and he confirms previously being treated for TB back in Morocco. ☐

4. A 36-year-old man is admitted via A&E with right-sided chest pain associated with SOB. There is no fever. O/E: Thin gentleman, smells of tobacco and alcohol. He is uncooperative to examination. Reduced breath sounds on the right side. Tender over the anterior chest wall. CXR: peripheral area of decreased lung markings on the right side. ☐

5. A 56-year-old insulin-dependent diabetic is admitted at the request of a concerned relative (a local doctor). He has been complaining of niggling chest pain for the past 2 days, with an associated feeling of SOB. O/E: No chest wall tenderness. Apyrexic. Nil adventitious sounds. HS I + II + 0. CXR: NAD. ECG: ST elevation 3 mm leads V4–V6 with T-wave inversion. Troponin 6.5 mg/L. ☐

4. **Theme: Shortness of breath**

(a) Pulmonary embolus
(b) Aortic stenosis
(c) Congestive cardiac failure
(d) Asthma
(e) Cryptogenic fibrosing alveolitis
(f) Pleural effusion
(g) Bronchial carcinoma
(h) COPD
(i) Right middle lobe pneumonia
(j) Pneumothorax

Instruction: *For each scenario described below, choose the SINGLE most likely diagnosis from the above list of options. Each option may be used once, more than once, or not at all.*

1. A 55-year-old baker is admitted with increasing shortness of breath over the past 6 weeks along with two syncopal episodes whilst at work. He suffered from asthma as a child. He admits to 20 pack years of smoking. Admission bloods, including d-dimer, are unremarkable. CXR: NAD. PEFR 450 L/min. ☐

2. A 32-year-old woman of childbearing age recently returned from a 2-month sabbatical in Thailand. She has been short of breath for the past week. O/E: Reduced air entry at the right middle and lower zones. No calf swelling. Oxygen saturations 92% (RA). D-dimer 0.45 mg/L, WCC 13.6×10^9/L. CXR: indistinct right heart border. ☐

3. A 61-year-old retired plumber is admitted with increasing shortness of breath over the past 2 months. He smokes 20 cigarettes a day. SOB is associated with mild pleuritic chest pain. O/E:

Reduced breath sounds at the left lower zone and decreased vocal resonance. CXR: loss of the left hemidiaphragm silhouette. Hb 12.6 g/dL, WCC 8.4 × 10⁹/L. ☐

4. A 24-year-old male Masters student is admitted to a district general hospital acutely SOB for the past day. He recalls a similar incident whilst a first year at University. He returned from a summer tour of Australasia 1 week ago. O/E: Oxygen saturations 93% (RA). Haemodynamically stable. Reduced breath sounds on left side and asymmetrical chest expansion. A medical student informs you 'the lungs look different' on the CXR. ☐

5. A 73-year-old former mill worker is admitted dyspnoeic with mild haemoptysis mixed with her sputum. She has had three previous admissions in the last 5 months with similar presentations. O/E: Thin, Grade 2 finger clubbing. Increased AP chest diameter with scattered wheeze and a few bibasal crepitations, right more than left. ABG (on 28% oxygen) PO_2 13.6 kPa, PCO_2 5.6 kPa. CXR: borderline cardiomegaly, blunted right costophrenic angle. Chronic inflammatory changes throughout and a bulky left hilum. ☐

5. Theme: Dysphagia

(a) Achalasia
(b) Motor neurone disease
(c) Oesophageal carcinoma
(d) Pharyngeal pouch
(e) Corrosive stricture
(f) Barrett's oesophagus
(g) Hiatus hernia
(h) Oesophageal varices
(i) Retrosternal thyroid
(j) Oesophageal web

Instruction: *For each scenario described below, choose the SINGLE most likely diagnosis from the above list of options. Each option may be used once, more than once, or not at all.*

1. A 68-year-old man attends outpatients with a 4-month history of increasing dysphagia and halitosis. His weight is stable as is his appetite, although he complains of bringing up undigested food at times. He also complains of the feeling of food getting stuck in his throat. He is teetotal and a non-smoker. He is otherwise well. Examination is unremarkable. ☐

2. A 52-year-old lady consults her GP with a 2-month history of increasing difficulty in swallowing. Her appetite is stable, although she is tired, but this has been ongoing for years. She has a history of microcytic anaemia and is on ferrous fumarate. She is a non-smoker and teetotal. She has never taken PPIs or H2 receptor antagonists. CXR: NAD. ☐

3. A 71-year-old former train driver is admitted to hospital with 2 stone in weight loss of unknown origin. On systematic questioning he admits to increasing difficulty with swallowing his favourite Sunday lunch and for the past 3 weeks has eaten only soup. He was previously a heavy drinker with 100 pack years of smoking. O/E: 4 cm hard, irregular hepar. Barium swallow demonstrated a stricture in the lower third of the oesophagus. ☐

4. A 65-year-old nun attends outpatients following a complaint to her GP of increasing difficulty swallowing. While awaiting this appointment she tells you she was admitted to hospital with a 'really bad' pneumonia on the right side of her chest for which she was given IV antibiotics. She is teetotal and a non-smoker. She has no medical history and on systemic review reveals no respiratory or neurological findings. O/E: NAD. CXR: widening of the mediastinum with an air fluid level and a resolving right basal pneumonia. ☐

5. A 36-year-old medical secretary visits surgical outpatients with a 2-month history of increasing difficulty swallowing and 1 stone in weight loss. She admits to poor sleep and occasional diarrhoea of late. O/E: Systolic flow murmur, weakness of the girdle muscles. No superficial neck swelling. CXR: superior mediastinal mass with mild tracheal shift. You are awaiting the results of FBP/U&E/TFTs and acetylcholine receptor antibodies. ☐

6. Theme: Appropriate imaging request

(a) PA chest radiograph
(b) CT chest
(c) HRCT chest
(d) VQ scan
(e) CT pulmonary angiogram
(f) MRI chest
(g) Lateral CXR
(h) Pulmonary angiogram
(i) PET scan (incorporating chest)
(j) Coronary angiography

Instruction: *Select the MOST APPROPRIATE INVESTIGATION from the list above for the clinical scenarios below. Each option may be used once, more than once, or not at all.*

1. A 43-year-old lady is referred from your rheumatology colleagues with a known diagnosis of rheumatoid disease. She has become increasingly SOB and has a dry cough. PFTs: FEV_1/FVC ratio normal. Reduced transfer factor. O/E: Fine bibasal creps. ☐

2. A 65-year-old man with a history of two myocardial infarcts is admitted acutely SOB. O/E: SpO_2 RA 88%, JVP raised 3 cm, 4th heart sound heard. Old ECHO report: 32% ejection fraction. ☐

3. A 52-year-old lady is admitted with a 2-day history of SOB, worse on breathing in, accompanied by haemoptysis. No past cardiac history. No recent foreign travel. Ex-smoker of 20 years. CXR: Emphysema. ECG: sinus tachycardia, RBBB. ☐

185

4. A 58-year-old lady is admitted with increasing SOB over the past 4 months. Over the past week she has had three incidences of haemoptysis. She has a history of 45 pack years, although doesn't smoke at present. In your opinion there is nothing obvious on the CXR. Admission bloods: Hb 9.3 g/dL, Na 128 mmol/L, K 3.9 Mmol/L, calcium 3.1 mmol/L, albumin 40 g/L, magnesium 0.99 mmol/L, phosphate 1.01 mmol/L. ☐

5. An otherwise fit 64-year-old man with known squamous cell bronchial carcinoma diagnosed at bronchoscopy. His FEV$_1$ is 2.5 litres. There was no evidence of hepatic or pulmonary metastases on CT. Calcium 2.4 Mmol/L, albumin 37 g/L, phosphate 1.02 Mmol/L. ☐

7. Theme: Neck lumps

(a) Thyroid nodule
(b) Branchial cyst
(c) Goitre
(d) Thyroglossal (duct) cyst
(e) Carotid body tumour
(f) Cystic hygroma
(g) Virchow's node (supraclavicular metastasis)
(h) Hodgkin's lymphoma
(i) Sebaceous cyst
(j) Parotid adenoma
(k) Anaplastic thyroid carcinoma

Instruction: *For each scenario described below, choose the SINGLE most likely diagnosis from the above list of options. Each option may be used once, more than once, or not at all.*

1. A 68-year-old retired seaman is admitted with weight loss of 1 stone over the past 4 months, reduced appetite and fatigue. Admission bloods: Hb 8.9 g/dL, MCV 69.5 fL, B$_{12}$ and folate normal. O/E: Fullness in the upper abdomen. ☐

2. An 18-year-old lady is admitted with a 3-month history of a swollen neck. She has no past medical history. She is unsure of any weight loss recently. Admission bloods reveal a normochromic anaemia. CXR: widened superior mediastinum. FNAC: Reed–Sternberg cells. ☐

3. A 21-year-old law student attends outpatients complaining of an enlarging lump in her neck. She had noticed it while preparing for an end of year formal. It is painless. O/E: 2 × 2 cm mobile mass at upper border of sternocleidomastoid in the anterior triangle. USS neck: cystic mass. ☐

4. A 53-year-old man is admitted for elective groin hernia repair. On assessment the houseman notes a 2 × 2 cm firm fixed mass in the anterior triangle on the left side. He undergoes a radiological procedure and the report states 'tumour blush'. ☐

5. A 23-year-old model attends the clinic conscious of a 2 × 3 cm mass in the anterior triangle of the neck. It is pain-free. It has grown over the past 4 months

and is mobile, firm but with no associated skin changes. It appears as a cystic hypoechoic mass on ultrasound. ☐

8. Theme: Headache

(a) Subarachnoid haemorrhage
(b) Migraine
(c) Skull fracture
(d) Tension headache
(e) Subdural haematoma
(f) Extradural haematoma
(g) Intracerebral haemorrhage
(h) Cerebral infarct
(i) Cerebral sinus thrombosis
(j) Idiopathic intracranial hypertension
(k) Viral encephalitis

Instruction: *For each scenario described below, choose the SINGLE most likely diagnosis from the above list of options. Each option may be used once, more than once, or not at all.*

1. An 18-year-old man was riding pillion on a motorbike without a helmet. At 50 mph he was seen to fall from the bike onto the road. At the scene he was found to have sustained multiple traumatic injuries to the thorax and limbs. His GCS was 8. His left pupil had a sluggish reaction to light. Work-up imaging included CT brain which revealed an elliptical, roughly 3 × 4 cm area of high attenuation peripherally. ☐

2. A 26-year-old postgraduate university student was admitted with headache and a 2-day history of recent alteration in her sense of smell. A mild pyrexia was noted by nursing staff. Lumbar puncture revealed a normal protein content, slightly raised leucocytes (lymphocytes predominant) and a normal plasma:CSF glucose ratio. CT brain was reported as normal. MRI brain (T2 weighted) revealed a slightly asymmetrical distribution of high signal within the temporal lobes bilaterally, more so on the right side. ☐

3. A 28-year-old mother of two is seen at outpatient clinic with a short history of headache—worse in the mornings and on stooping to attend to her young children. She has no past medical history although she is attending a dietitian-led weight loss clinic. Her only medication is the OCP as she does not wish for further children at present. O/E: Bilateral papilloedema. CT brain: normal. ☐

4. A 73-year-old lady who lives alone was found by her neighbour to be behaving oddly of late and more unsteady on her feet over the past couple of weeks. She has a medical history that includes hypertension, atrial fibrillation, previous THR and Parkinson's disease. O/E: She is disorientated in time and place. Her mood was fluctuant. CT brain: low attenuation crescenteric region adjacent to the right temporal bone. ☐

5. A 28-year-old working mother re-attended outpatient clinic complaining of a 9-month history of headache. They are now occurring around three times a week, mostly on weekdays, and were partially responsive to codeine-based analgesics. The headache is felt across the whole head, with no visual disturbance or nausea. Complete neurological examination was normal. CT brain had been done at her second visit, largely on patient request for peace of mind and was reported as normal. ☐

6. A 76-year-old lady was admitted to A&E following a collapse at home. She lives alone and was found by her daughter on the bedroom floor. Her past medical history consists of angina and peripheral vascular disease. Skull x-ray taken initially was normal. O/E: Right-sided weakness. Speech was normal. CT brain (at 24 hours): low attenuation area in the region of left internal capsule with adjacent oedema. ☐

9. Theme: Joint pain

(a) Rheumatoid arthritis
(b) Psoriatic arthritis
(c) Ankylosing spondylitis
(d) Reactive arthritis
(e) Pseudogout
(f) Gout
(g) Septic joint
(h) Bone infarct
(i) Pathological fracture
(j) SLE

Instruction: *For each scenario described below, choose the SINGLE most likely diagnosis from the above list of options. Each option may be used once, more than once, or not at all.*

1. A 65-year-old lady presented to her GP with an acutely swollen left knee. She had no chronic illnesses and is on no medications. On examination there was evidence of an effusion. It was painful on palpation. All other joints were unremarkable. Her old notes reveal a similar problem in the past—an x-ray was taken previously. It reported chondrocalcinosis of the left knee. ☐

2. A 9-year-old child presented to A&E with a 16-hour history of a red, hot, tender, right knee. On examination the right knee was warm to the touch and exquisitely painful. The knee was aspirated but no crystals were noted. WCC was elevated. Ultrasound demonstrated a large effusion. No bony erosion seen. ☐

3. A 45-year-lady was seen at the outpatient clinic with a year-long history of pain in the small joints of hands, feet and the left wrist. She complained of stiffness on waking in the mornings. Her GP had undertaken a number of blood tests: ESR and CRP were elevated, ANA and RF were reported as within normal range. O/E: Warmth and swelling over multiple MCP and PIP joints bilaterally in keeping with active synovitis. No rash or nodules noted. Radiographs of hands and feet: periarticular erosions at right 3rd and 4th and left 3rd MCP joints. Soft tissue swelling noted adjacent to multiple MCP and PIP joints in both hands. ☐

4. A 39-year-old gentleman was referred by his GP with lower back and joint pains. He had not sustained any injury and gives an 8-month history of lower back pain and more recently discomfort of the wrists and several fingers in the left hand. O/E: Swelling and tenderness of the 2nd, 3rd and 4th DIP joints in the left hand. Both wrists tender and reduced range of active movement. Inflammatory markers were raised. ANA and RF negative. Radiographs of hands reveal normal bone density. Erosions at the DIP joints correlate with clinical findings. ☐

5. A 35-year-old lady is admitted to hospital with a number of symptoms, including painful joints, tiredness and a rash. This has caused her to be off work for the last 6 weeks. O/E: Pale. Apyrexic. A number of small joints of both hands are tender to touch. Admission bloods reveal ESR 67 mm/hr, CRP 8 ng/L, Hb 10.2 g/dL, WCC 2.4×10^9/L. Radiographs and ultrasound of the joints were normal. ☐

6. A 49-year-old man with a history of HOCM and Grade 3 heart failure is admitted to cardiology with acute pulmonary oedema. ECHO confirms pre-existing disease and an estimated ejection fraction of 24%. He receives treatment in addition to his regular cardiac medications. On day 4 of his admission he complains of a red, hot, swollen right elbow. A cannula is sited in his left forearm for IV medication administration. X-ray reveals soft tissue swelling. ☐

7. A 47-year-old man is currently an inpatient in the hepatology unit which he has attended on a number of occasions in the past 5 years. He has been a diabetic for the past 4 years. He develops an acutely sore right knee. It is hot, red and swollen, both subjectively and objectively. Ultrasound of the knee confirms an effusion. It is aspirated, the results of which shows no growth. ☐

10. Theme: Principles of radiology

(a) MRI
(b) Ultrasound
(c) HRCT
(d) Helical CT
(e) PET imaging
(f) Barium contrast studies
(g) Fluoroscopy
(h) Mammography
(i) VQ scan
(j) Radio-labelled white cell scan

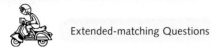

Instruction: *Select the MOST APPROPRIATE INVESTIGATION from the list above for the clinical scenarios below. Each option may be used once, more than once, or not at all.*

1. Imaging modality of choice for the assessment of sufferers of chronic pulmonary sarcoidosis. ☐

2. Imaging investigation(s) associated with the assessment of functional rather than structural disease. ☐

3. Radiological investigations without requirement for radiation exposure procedures. ☐

4. Procedure(s) with which attenuation value ranges are given the term Hounsfield units. ☐

5. Procedure with which the generation of an image is produced in part by alteration in the shape of a piezoelectric crystal. ☐

6. Imaging modality which best demonstrates demyelination within the cerebral white matter. ☐

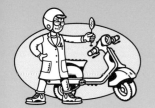
To complete these questions please refer to the images indicated.

1. **Pneumonia (see Fig. 19.11b, page 109)**

    (a) What can be observed on this chest radiograph?
    (b) What do you understand by the loss of the silhouette sign?
    (c) Which subtype of this condition is highly associated with HIV/AIDS?
    (d) What is an air bronchogram?

2. **Pleural effusion (see Fig. 19.21, page 112)**

    (a) What can be observed on this chest radiograph?
    (b) What other imaging modality can be of use to confirm the diagnosis of this complaint?
    (c) What else may be seen on a chest radiograph with a very large type of this condition?
    (d) Suggest underlying conditions responsible for this chest radiograph appearance

3. **Pneumothorax (see Fig. 19.13, page 110)**

    (a) What can be observed on this chest radiograph?
    (b) Which type of radiograph makes this condition easier to diagnose and why?
    (c) Why does the radiograph appear darker at the edges?
    (d) What additional signs may be seen if this radiograph was of a tension pneumothorax?
    (e) How would you treat this condition?

4. **Congestive cardiac failure (see Fig. 20.5, page 116)**

    (a) What can be observed on this chest radiograph?
    (b) What other imaging may be useful in the management of this patient?
    (c) What are the classic radiographic features of this condition?
    (d) Explain why upper lobe diversion occurs
    (e) What respiratory condition may be confused with this condition by radiological appearance?

5. **Peripheral vascular disease (see Fig. 20.9, page 117)**

    (a) What do you understand by the term 'digital subtraction angiography'?
    (b) What do you see on this image?
    (c) What options does an interventional radiologist have to treat this condition?
    (d) What do you understand by negative and positive contrast agents?
    (e) If this patient had renal impairment, how would this influence your choice of contrast agent?

6. **Oesophageal carcinoma (see Fig. 21.7, page 116)**

    (a) What can be seen on this image?
    (b) Describe how this procedure is performed.
    (c) What kind of stricture do you associate with shouldering and why does it occur?
    (d) What further imaging would you request given this diagnosis?
    (e) In which part of the oesophagus is this condition most commonly seen?

7. **Pneumoperitoneum (see Fig. 21.9, page 126)**

    (a) What can be observed on this image?
    (b) Give some reasons for why the findings are present
    (c) How could this appear on a supine film?
    (d) What do you understand by Chilaiditi's syndrome with relevance to this condition?
    (e) With reference to 'abnormal gas', with what condition would you see the double bubble sign?

8. **Large bowel obstruction (with CRC on barium enema) (see Fig. 21.22, page 130)**

    (a) What can be observed on this image?
    (b) How does one distinguish large and small bowel on a plain radiograph?
    (c) How does this same condition appear on a radiograph when it affects the small bowel?
    (d) What do you understand by the term 'cut-off sign'?
    (e) What other imaging may be necessary?

9. **Osteoarthritis of the hip (see Fig. 23.23, page 150)**

    (a) What can you observe on this image?
    (b) What are the four classic radiological signs of this condition?
    (c) Why do osteophytes form?
    (d) What causes of this condition are you aware of?

10. **Breast carcinoma (see Fig. 20.18, page 120)**

    (a) What do you call these two radiographic views?
    (b) What can you observe on this image?
    (c) What further imaging would you request given the likely diagnosis?
    (d) How would your approach to imaging change if this lady was less than 40 years of age?
    (e) Which growing group of patients require special films on screening mammography?

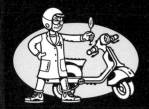

1. (a) T
   (b) T
   (c) T
   (d) T
   (e) F—There is no strong association between antibiotic allergy and IV contrast agents

2. (a) T
   (b) T
   (c) F—Cryptogenic fibrosing alveolitis affects the lower zones predominantly
   (d) T
   (e) T

3. (a) F—CXR can be suggestive of bronchial carcinoma but is not pathognomonic
   (b) T
   (c) F—Liver and adrenal glands are routinely imaged for tumour staging but not the brain
   (d) F—Alkaline phosphatase can be raised for reasons other than bronchial carcinoma with metastases and in itself is not an indication for a bone scan
   (e) T

4. (a) T
   (b) F—Bone cysts are a feature of osteoarthritis, not rheumatoid arthritis
   (c) T
   (d) F—The MCP and PIP joints are classically involved in rheumatoid arthritis
   (e) F—The 'pencil in cup' deformity is a feature of psoriatic arthritis

5. (a) T
   (b) F—Pleural plaques are seen in less than 50% of those exposed to asbestos
   (c) T
   (d) F—Pleural effusions can occur, but are not common
   (e) F—Pleural thickening commonly occurs

6. (a) F—Less than 7 mm is within normal range
   (b) T
   (c) T
   (d) F—Only 10–15% of gallstones are seen on AXR; 80% refers to renal calculi
   (e) T

7. (a) F—MRI is not contraindicated in welders, but orbital x-rays are required of anyone (welders especially high risk) who could have a foreign body in the eye
   (b) T
   (c) F—MRI makes use of the properties of hydrogen ions, not helium ions
   (d) F—MRI has no radiation dose
   (e) T

8. (a) F—Microcalcification can occur in benign and malignant breast disease
   (b) F—50–70-year-old women are invited to screening
   (c) F—Two projections are taken at screening: craniocaudal and oblique
   (d) T
   (e) F—A spiculated lesion is characteristic of a malignant mass

9. (a) T
   (b) T
   (c) F—Small bowel enema has a higher radiation dose than small bowel series
   (d) T
   (e) T

10. (a) F—Ultrasound of the neck is not essential as it does not reliably distinguish malignant from benign thyroid masses
    (b) T
    (c) F—A solid lesion is malignant in only 10% of cases and a malignant lesion is not always solid
    (d) T
    (e) T

11 (a) F—Biopsy of a testicular lesion is contraindicated as the tumour may seed along the track of the biopsy
    (b) T
    (c) T
    (d) F—Left sided varicocoeles are associated with renal cell carcinoma
    (e) T

12. (a) T
    (b) T
    (c) F—A mismatched defect of perfusion and ventilation is characteristic on VQ scan
    (d) F—Hyperexpansion is not a feature of pulmonary embolus
    (e) T

13. (a) F—A sentinel loop is rarely seen (and often retrospectively!)
(b) F—A pseudocyst is best seen on ultrasound or CT of the abdomen
(c) T
(d) F—Pneumoperitoneum is not a feature of acute pancreatitis
(e) F—CT is more reliable in assessing for pancreatic oedema; ultrasound is less useful due to bowel gas often obscuring the pancreas

14. (a) F—The right heart border is obscured with right middle lobe consolidation; the right superior mediastinum is obscured with right upper lobe consolidation
(b) T
(c) F—Left lower lobe collapse obscures the left hemidiaphragm and produces the 'sail sign'
(d) F—Right middle lobe consolidation obscures the right heart border; the right hemidiaphragm silhouette is lost in right lower lobe consolidation
(e) T

15. (a) T
(b) T
(c) T
(d) T
(e) F—Triple therapy consists of clinical assessment, pathology (FNAC and/or biopsy) and imaging

16. (a) T
(b) F—Periarticular erosions are a feature of rheumatoid arthritis
(c) T
(d) F—Periarticular osteopenia is a feature of rheumatoid arthritis
(e) F—Osteoclasts are new bone-forming cells and are not seen on plain radiograph. Osteophytes are seen on radiographs

17. (a) T
(b) F—This is not reliable; a DEXA scan is required
(c) T
(d) T
(e) T

18. (a) F—Lytic metastases are commoner than sclerotic metastases
(b) F—Sclerotic metastases most commonly arise from prostatic (not testicular) tumours
(c) T
(d) F—Lytic metastases are seen as destructive areas of radiolucency
(e) T

19. (a) T
(b) F—Not a feature – the cysts do not calcify in APKD
(c) F—Hyperparathyroidism causes calcium deposition, not hypoparathyroidism
(d) T
(e) T

20. (a) T
(b) T
(c) F—Hyperparathyroidism may give rise to CXR calcification but not hyperthyroidism
(d) T
(e) T

21. (a) T
(b) F—One AXR is equivalent to 35 CXRs
(c) F—CT scan of chest is equivalent to 2.5 years of background radiation
(d) F—A barium enema is equivalent to 350 CXRs
(e) T

22. (a) F—Both sigmoid and caecal volvuli are more common than gastric
(b) F—Faecal peritonitis can occur, especially if untreated, but is not common
(c) T
(d) F
(e) F—Intussusception is telescoping of the bowel within itself. It is another cause of bowel obstruction like volvulus

23. (a) T
(b) T
(c) F—Upper lobe diversion is a feature of cardiac failure
(d) F—There is no recognized association between heart size on CXR and ejection fraction
(e) F—TOE is more beneficial for assessment of valves, not left ventricular function

24. (a) T
(b) T
(c) T
(d) F—HRCT is the imaging modality of choice for interstitial lung disease
(e) F—CT is not contraindicated in patients with pacemakers, although some artefact will be produced, reducing imaging quality in adjacent areas

25. (a) F—Long stenoses are less suitable for a stent to be placed across
(b) F—There is no good evidence of angioplasty being superior to surgery for distal disease
(c) F—More than 90% of patients will receive an iodine-containing contrast agent
(d) T
(e) F—Angioplasty limb loss rate is around 0.5% and less in most centres

26. (a) T
(b) T
(c) T
(d) T
(e) F—Gas is not seen within the biliary tree in necrotizing enterocolitis. It can be seen in the portal vein.

27. (a) T
    (b) F—10–15% of gallstones are seen on AXR
    (c) F—Gallstones are seen as high density structures on CT; they are seen as filling defects in ERCP
    (d) T
    (e) T

28. (a) T
    (b) F—There is no cavitation with pulmonary contusion, however pulmonary infarcts may cavitate
    (c) T
    (d) T
    (e) T

29. (a) T
    (b) F—Pneumothorax is best seen on an expiratory film
    (c) F—not if small
    (d) F—A tension pneumothorax causes diaphragmatic depression, not elevation
    (e) T

30. (a) F—The kidneys are situated between the T12 and L2 vertebrae
    (b) T
    (c) T
    (d) F—Biliary gas is always pathological
    (e) F—The abdominal aorta outline is only seen when calcified

31. (a) T
    (b) F—Loss of the right heart border indicates right middle lobe consolidation
    (c) T
    (d) F—Between five and seven anterior ribs should be visible on CXR and up to 10 posterior ribs in the mid-clavicular line
    (e) T

32. (a–e) All true

33. (a) T
    (b) T
    (c) T
    (d) F—Prominence of the left atrial appendage is a feature of mitral stenosis
    (e) F—The aortic knuckle is normal

34. (a) F—Fibrosis from tuberculosis is typically in the upper zones
    (b) T
    (c) T
    (d) T
    (e) F—Lung capacity is either normal or reduced in tuberculosis

35. (a) T
    (b) T
    (c) F—Reticulonodular shadowing is seen with progression to honeycomb lung but not a complete whiteout
    (d) F—ARDS causes diffuse alveolar shadowing
    (e) T

36. (a) T
    (b) F—A mediastinal mass can cause tracheal shift, but this is not common
    (c) T
    (d) T
    (e) T

37. (a) F—50% of sarcoidosis sufferers have bilateral hilar lymphadenopathy on CXR
    (b) F—Hilar enlargement in pulmonary hypertension is due to enlarged pulmonary vessels, not lymphadenopathy
    (c) T
    (d) T
    (e) F—ARDS does not cause radiographic evidence of hilar node disease

38. (a) F—Age and lifestyle are not indications for AAA screening at present, although they are risk factors
    (b) F—Screening is done 6 monthly for those with a 4.6–5.5 cm AAA
    (c) T
    (d) T
    (e) T

39. (a) F—TIAs could relate to symptoms from ischaemia to the posterior circulation in which case carotid artery imaging is not useful
    (b) T
    (c) F—A patient must be symptomatic and have a stenosis of greater than 70% to be a surgical candidate
    (d) F—Only angiography should not be undertaken due to the risk–benefit ratio of this investigation
    (e) T

40. (a) T
    (b) T
    (c) F—Coarctation may occur in the absence of cardiac failure, especially if the patient is young
    (d) F—Classically occurs just distal to the left subclavian artery
    (e) F—There is no association between coarctation and pulmonary hypertension (of which peripheral pruning is a feature)

41. (a) F—Upper zone fibrosis (and hence retraction) causes tenting of the diaphragm
    (b) T
    (c) F—Bleomycin causes lower zone fibrosis
    (d) T
    (e) T

42. (a) T
    (b) T
    (c) F—Blood is shunted from the right to the left atrium, causing right ventricular hypertrophy
    (d) F—There is a boot-shaped heart and pulmonary oligaemia
    (e) F—The aortic knuckle is not affected in PDA

43. (a) T
 (b) F—A renal pelvis diameter of >1 cm is significant
 (c) T
 (d) F—Two-thirds (66%) of cases will have VUR
 (e) F—CT scans are rarely used; extracapsular spread or unusual organisms are indications for CT

44. (a) F—All should have passed meconium by 48 hours
 (b) F—The commonest site is the rectosigmoid region
 (c) F—10–15% of neonates with CF present with meconium ileus
 (d) T
 (e) F—'Double bubble' is seen in infants with duodenal atresia

45. (a) T
 (b) F—The femoral head ossifies at 4–6 months old
 (c) F—The cause is unknown
 (d) T
 (e) T

46. (a) T
 (b) F—The slip is posteromedial
 (c) T
 (d) T
 (e) F—The condition is bilateral in one-third of cases

47. (a) T
 (b) T
 (c) F—Duodenal atresia is distal to the ampulla
 (d) F—Maternal oligohydramnios is a risk factor
 (e) F—Right-to-left shunts produce cyanosis

48. (a) T
 (b) F—Non-contrast scans are more sensitive in diagnosing haemorrhage
 (c) T
 (d) F—Middle cerebral artery aneurysms rupture into the sylvian fissure
 (e) F—Hemiparesis is a common presenting complaint, not paraparesis

49. (a) F—CT is the investigation of choice
 (b) F—GCS less than 12
 (c) T
 (d) T
 (e) T

50. (a) F—SAH produces hyperdensities in the subarachnoid spaces
 (b) F—The commonest cause is an aneurysm
 (c) F—Colloid cysts obstruct the foramen of Monroe
 (d) F—Infratentorial location is the commonest location
 (e) F—Evening presentation suggests a benign tension headache

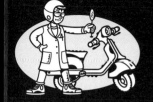

SAQ Answers

1. Calcification on an abdominal radiograph (AXR) can be normal or abnormal. Abnormal calcification may indicate underlying pathology, such as an abdominal aortic aneurysm, or be the pathology in itself, such as a renal calculus.

   Non-pathological calcification includes costocalcinosis, calcified mesenteric lymph nodes, prostate calcification and pelvic phleboliths. Calcification that indicates pathology includes pancreatic, renal (nephrocalcinosis), arterial calcification. Nephrocalcinosis involves the renal parenchymal tissue, occurring in conditions such as hyperparathyroidism, medullary sponge kidney, sarcoidosis and renal tubular acidosis.

   Calcification, which is the pathology in itself, consists mostly of various calculi. Biliary (10–20% seen), renal (80%), bladder and appendicolith. Rarely a porcelain gallbladder or a teratoma is observed on the plain abdominal radiograph.

2. The most commonly requested imaging investigation and hence the most commonly requested radiologically based exam question is to present/interpret a chest radiograph. Cardiorespiratory disease accounts for a significant proportion of acute medical admissions and consequently findings on CXR often dictate medical management.

   The film should be fully illuminated on a light box, with as little finger contact as possible, not least in the heat of an exam, to avoid sticky fingerprints! As with any film, if there is two of anything, always use these for comparison.

   Initially comment on the film specifics. The exact details of projection (AP, PA, semi-erect), the type of film (CXR, AXR) and the date the film was taken. It may be part of a series and thus other films are needed for accurate comparison and comment. The patient details are added to the introductory statement, chiefly the name and age and perhaps on occasion the location (e.g. cardiac ICU).

   Technical assessment follows, with assessment of rotation, inspiration and penetration (RIP). There should be equidistance between the spinous processes and the medial ends of the clavicles. Change in this implies rotation and thus alteration in the dimensions of other structures. Ten posterior or greater than five to seven anterior ribs should be visible in the mid-clavicular line. The thoracic vertebrae should be clearly seen at the mid-thoracic spine if properly penetrated.

   You are now in the position to look for pathology in a systematic fashion, viewing the following areas: heart, lungs, mediastinum and pleura, bones and soft tissues, review areas.

   There are three key aspects to the cardiac evaluation: heart size (cardiothoracic ratio), heart borders and the pulmonary vascularity. The last reflects the pulmonary wedge pressure which increases in cardiac failure. To review pulmonary and mediastinal structures, check the trachea is central, the size, shape and level of the hila, the lungs, comparing one side with the other. There are four key points to review with regard to the diaphragm: its level, shape, the presence of any subdiaphragmatic gas/collection and whether the costophrenic angles are blunted. Finally, view the pleura for any thickening or evidence of a pneumothorax.

   With regard to the bones and soft tissues, check the ribs, clavicle and humerus on both sides for fractures and metastatic involvement. You may also note any other generalized bone diseases. Surgical emphysema and soft tissue masses may be observed. Breast shadows are important in women—the loss of one suggesting previous mastectomy for breast carcinoma.

   Don't forget to comment on any artefactual findings—pacemakers, sternotomy wires, coronary stents being just a few.

3. Abdominal aortic aneurysms can present in four ways: following a rupture (emergency), with mild symptoms (subacute), coincidently on clinical examination and following imaging investigations for other indications. This is likely to be an AXR, ultrasound abdomen or CT abdomen.

   Acute ruptures should be in theatre, not the radiology department, but those with subacute symptoms or a suspicion on clinical examination should initially proceed to an ultrasound of the abdomen. It is safe, easy and quick, and has no radiation exposure. Size, wall thickness and any evidence of 'leakage' can be detected. The results of this and patient factors will dictate if further imaging by contrast enhanced CT abdomen is indicated.

   A key element of elective AAA management is risk–benefit analysis with regard to surgery. For this reason surveillance of AAAs of 3.5–5.5 cm by ultrasound is commonplace: 3.5–4.5 cm AAAs are followed by yearly USS, 4.6–5.5 cm are followed 6-monthly and those greater than 5.5 cm considered for repair—either open or by endovascular stenting (EVAR trials 1 and 2*). An AAA that is increasing in

*EVAR trial participants. Endovascular aneurysm repair versus open repair in patients with abdominal aortic aneurysm (EVAR trial 1): randomised controlled trial. Lancet 2005;365:2179–86; EVAR trial participants. Endovascular aneurysm repair and outcome in patients unfit for open repair of abdominal aortic aneurysm (EVAR trial 2): randomised controlled trial. Lancet 2005;365:2187–92

size by more than 1 cm a year also requires closer monitoring. Recent studies[†] suggest that in future a national screening programme of all men over 65 would save lives and be cost effective.

Before elective surgery, a contrast enhanced CT should be performed. The exact dimensions of the aneurysm, most importantly the diameter, can be delineated. The length of the aneurysm neck and the thickness of the aneurysm wall can also be evaluated. A thick wall suggests an inflammatory aneurysm. Perhaps most essential for the surgeon is the relationship of the aneurysm to the renal vessels; those that are infrarenal (80%) are the most amenable to surgery. With modern multislice CT, 3D reconstruction can be undertaken. Any involvement of distal iliac vessels is also useful to know.

4. There are a number of valuable investigations available for the imaging of the jaundiced patient. These should be targeted to clinical suspicions and requested in a logical sequence. The modalities used may also be influenced by radiation dose, ease of performing the test, local availability and the patient's condition.

Following clinical examination and biochemical assessment (liver function tests), an ultrasound scan of the abdomen is a good starting point, not least as the two commonest causes of obstructive jaundice are biliary disease and pancreatic carcinoma (although the pancreas may be obscured by bowel gas on ultrasound). There may have been an AXR performed on admission. This is more often than not normal, but may show gallstones or biliary gas, depending on the cause of the jaundice. Ultrasound essentially distinguishes if the cause of the jaundice is obstructive or non-obstructive (hepatic). A gallstone in the common hepatic duct with proximal dilatation would suggest cholelithiasis. The biliary tree, especially if intervention of some description is likely (e.g. stone removal), can be explored using ERCP and PTC.

MRCP is of growing value in imaging the biliary tree; however, no intervention is possible with this modality. ERCP remains the gold standard, despite its well-recognized complications, such as acute pancreatitis. It will identify calculi, which may be removed at the same time, demonstrate a stricture and can be used for taking pathological specimens or stent insertion. If ERCP is not suitable due to the patient's condition or is technically difficult, PTC can be performed if calculi or strictures are suspected in the upper common bile duct. PTC also permits biopsy and insertion of a drain—a useful procedure in those requiring palliation. Those suspected of having a pancreatic mass will benefit from CT of the abdomen.

[†]Multicentre Aneurysm Screening Study Group. Multicentre aneurysm screening study (MASS): cost effectiveness analysis of screening for abdominal aortic aneurysms based on four year results from randomised controlled trial. BMJ 2002;325:1135–8

5. It is important to be able to distinguish a mechanical small bowel obstruction from one involving the large bowel. Likewise, distinguishing between these and an ileus or pseudo-obstruction is important in the management of these patients.

In small bowel obstruction the loops tend to be centrally placed and less than 5 cm in diameter (but greater than 3 cm); there are usually multiple bowel loops and the valvulae conniventes can be observed. No gas can be seen within the large bowel. Contrast this with large bowel obstruction where there are usually few bowel loops, greater than 5 cm in diameter at the periphery of the film. There are haustra evident and a clear cut-off point identified.

Although adhesions from previous surgery is the commonest cause of bowel obstruction, it is important in all over-50 year olds to rule out a colorectal carcinoma, i.e. an intraluminal cause of the obstruction. Bowel obstruction need not always be absolute—subacute (perhaps better named partial) obstruction is a common cause of admission to a surgical ward and often responds well to conservative treatment.

6. The finding of a pulmonary mass on CXR, especially in smokers over 40 years of age, should always arouse suspicion of a malignant focal lesion—either primary or secondary. How it is investigated in the first instance depends on the clinical presentation, local protocols and the availability of competing investigative techniques. CT chest and upper abdomen (to include the liver and adrenal glands) is likely to be required. If either initially or after CT the likelihood of a bronchial carcinoma is high, bronchoscopy with biopsies and washings will aid confirmation and subtyping. The subtype is important in bronchial carcinoma as it dictates management. One may also consider in selected cases the merits of a radio-isotope bone scan for bony metastases (bony pain). CT brain for evidence of cerebral metastases is not routinely performed in most centres. PET/CT (where available) has a pre-eminent position in tumour staging.

7. Patients symptomatic with peripheral vascular disease suffer from intermittent claudication—the equivalent of 'angina of the legs'—the underlying process being essentially the same, i.e. stenosed arteries secondary to atherosclerosis. Ankle brachial pressure index (ABPI) is a useful initial test as it is non-invasive. The gold standard for assessing the true nature and degree of stenosis is by catheter angiography as this will delineate the location, number and extent of any stenoses and their amenability to intervention. However, many centres now routinely use magnetic resonance angiography (MRA) for diagnostic workup. Management options include both conservative and interventional—either endovascular or surgical. Conservative treatment entails reducing cardiovascular risk factors and encouraging the development of a collateral

circulation. Intervention offers bypass surgery and, from a radiologist's perspective, angioplasty, with or without the placement of an endoluminal stent.

8. The investigation of a breast lump is based around the accepted practice of triple assessment. Imaging is one component of this assessment and comprises mammography and/or ultrasound. Standard procedure is for a craniocaudal and an oblique mammogram to be taken. Signs suggestive of malignancy include microcalcification, an abnormal contour to the breast border and spiculation (a star-like appearance). Microcalcification in itself is not diagnostic of a breast carcinoma—it can occur in other benign breast conditions such as fat necrosis. In the under 35 year olds, mammography is of more limited value. This is because the premenopausal breast has a greater glandular component which is of a greater density than fat and similar in density to a tumour mass. It is therefore difficult to identify a tumour mass. In younger patients ultrasound is commonly used, as it is in those thought to have a cystic lump. Ultrasound demonstrates cysts well and can be used to aid drainage.

   Imaging also plays an important role in guided biopsies, usually by ultrasound, although on occasion guide wires are placed stereotactically for surgeons to localize a lump.

9. A chest radiograph, like other plain films, demonstrates only four natural densities: black for gas, white for calcified structures, grey for soft tissues and darker grey for fat. This reflects the amount of radiation absorbed by structures of varying density and thus the amount that reaches the x-ray plate or digital receptor. When two structures of a great difference in density are adjacent to one another, a distinct border—or silhouette—is formed (e.g. the lung apex and the clavicle). The lung is of low density so few x-rays are absorbed and the film is black, whereas the clavicle, containing high density material, absorbs more x-rays so the film appears white as fewer x-rays expose the plate. This large contrast is the silhouette. This phenomenon is of great value in comparing lung tissue adjacent to denser structures, chiefly the heart and diaphragms:
   - Left upper lobe: aortic knuckle
   - Lingula: left heart border
   - Left lower lobe: left hemidiaphragm
   - Right upper lobe: right superior mediastinum
   - Right middle lobe: right heart border
   - Right lower lobe: right hemidiaphragm.

   For example, if there is infective consolidation of the left lower lobe the silhouette formed between this lobe of the lung and the left hemidiaphragm will be lost, i.e. the clear distinct outline of the hemidiaphragm is obscured (see Ch. 1).

10. Severe mitral stenosis invariably arises secondary to rheumatic fever, giving rise to some distinctive radiological signs on CXR.
   - Double right heart border: Left atrial enlargement occurs secondary to a stenosed valve as back pressure causes atrial enlargement. This forms a double border to the right side of the heart—one the normal right ventricle wall and the other the left atrial wall.
   - Splaying of the carina (greater than 90°): The enlarged left atrium pushes on the adjacent trachea causing it to splay.
   - Prominence of the left atrial appendage on the left side of the heart on CXR: This follows left atrial enlargement.
   - Valve calcification: A stenosed rheumatic valve can become calcified as can a markedly enlarged left atrial wall on occasion.
   - Heart failure signs: As the heart can begin to fail secondary to the mitral stenosis, all the radiological signs of heart failure may be apparent: cardiomegaly, pleural effusions, Kerley B lines, upper lobe venous diversion and interstitial oedema.

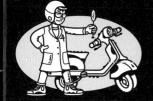

EMQ Answers

1. Theme: Altered bowel habit
1. Diverticulitis (g)
2. Irritable bowel syndrome (d)
3. Crohn's disease (b)
4. Ulcerative colitis (a)
5. Colorectal carcinoma (c)

2. Theme: Jaundice
1. Pancreatic carcinoma (d)
2. Hepatocellular carcinoma (c)
3. Chronic pancreatitis (i)
4. Gallbladder carcinoma (e)
5. Liver abscess (j)

3. Theme: Chest pain
1. Pulmonary embolus (b)
2. GORD (secondary to NSAID) (d)
3. Pericarditis (c)
4. Rib fracture (with associated pneumothorax) (e)
5. Myocardial infarct (lateral) (a)

4. Theme: Shortness of breath
1. Aortic stenosis (b)
2. Right middle lobe pneumonia (i)
3. Pleural effusion (f)
4. Spontaneous pneumothorax (j)
5. Bronchial carcinoma (g)

5. Theme: Dysphagia
1. Pharyngeal pouch (d)
2. Oesophageal web (j)
3. Oesophageal carcinoma (c)
4. Achalasia (a)
5. Retrosternal thyroid (i)

6. Theme: Appropriate Imaging request
1. HRCT (c) (This lady most likely has interstitial lung disease)
2. CXR (a) (This gentleman is in acute LVF)
3. CTPA (e) (This history is suggestive of a PE)
4. CT chest (b) (This lady most likely has a bronchial carcinoma)
5. PET scan (i) (This gentleman is a potential surgical candidate)

7. Theme: Neck lumps
1. Virchow's node (g)
2. Hodgkin's lymphoma (h)
3. Branchial cyst (b)
4. Carotid body tumour (e)
5. Sebaceous cyst (i)

8. Theme: Headache
1. Extradural haematoma (f)
2. Viral encephalitis (herpes simplex) (k)
3. Idiopathic intracranial hypertension (j)
4. Subdural haematoma (chronic) (e)
5. Tension headache (d)
6. Cerebral infarct (h)

9. Theme: Joint pain
1. Pseudogout (e)
2. Septic joint (g)
3. Rheumatoid arthritis (sero-negative) (a)
4. Psoriatic arthritis (b)
5. SLE (j)
6. Gout (f)
7. Pseudogout (as part of haemochromatosis) (e)

10. Theme: Principles of radiology
1. HRCT (c)
2. PET imaging (e), VQ scan (i) and radio-labelled white cell scan (j)
3. MRI (a) and ultrasound (b)
4. HRCT (c) and helical CT (d)
5. Ultrasound (b)
6. MRI (a)

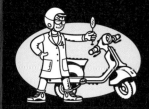

OSCE Answers

1. Pneumonia

(a) There is an area of increased radio-opacity in the left lower lobe of the lung. There is a loss of the silhouette between the left lobe of the lung and the left hemidiaphragm. This suggests increased density of the lung secondary to consolidation.

(b) The density on a plain radiograph is reflective of the density of the structures on it. Bone which is very dense absorbs most x-rays and so less of the film is irradiated, giving a white appearance. The lung, being chiefly gas, absorbs few x-rays, causing blackness as most x-rays expose the film. Therefore, if two structures of different densities are close together, a silhouette (distinct border) is observed. If the density of one of these structures changes, as with lung consolidation, the silhouette is lost. For example, in right middle lobe consolidation the right heart border silhouette is lost.

(c) *Pneumocystis jiroveci* (formerly *P. carinii*) pneumonia is associated with the immunosuppressed state of HIV/AIDS.

(d) When the lung tissue becomes consolidated by infection, the bronchioles initially stay patent, with gas retained within. However, the surrounding tissue is likely to be consolidated so these small circular or linear areas of radiolucency stand out from the surrounding parenchyma.

2. Pleural effusion

(a) There is loss of the left costophrenic angle (angle between the diaphragm and lateral border of the chest). It appears radio-opaque (white), suggesting fluid/soft tissue within the thorax. At the lateral limit of this radio-opacity there is a meniscus (the density tapers up at the edge), suggesting fluid. This represents a pleural effusion.

(b) On occasion there may be indication for an ultrasound scan to identify fluid within the pleural space, perhaps with a view to localization for aspiration purposes.

(c) In cases of large pleural effusion there may be mediastinal shift and deviation of the trachea away from the effusion. Often, however, associated collapse of the lung masks the mass effect of the effusion.

(d) Pleural effusions may be unilateral or bilateral, large or small, exudate or transudate. Causes of transudates include heart failure, hepatic and renal failure and hypoalbuminaemia. Exudates are caused by infection, primary and secondary malignancy of the lung, a pulmonary embolus and pulmonary infarction among others. Generally, exudates are due to localized causes and transudates to systemic causes.

3. Pneumothorax

(a) A right lung edge can be seen. Peripheral to this it is radiolucent as there is no lung tissue present.

(b) An erect expiratory film. This helps accentuate the appearance of gas within the pleural space due to a relatively increased pleural pressure within the thorax on expiration.

(c) It is darker at the edge as there is no lung present, the intrapleural space containing only gas. Hence, pulmonary vascular markings/bronchioles are not evident. The pulmonary vascular markings are what normally give the lung its characteristic appearance.

(d) A tension pneumothorax is a medical emergency. If clinical suspicions are of this then one should not wait for radiographic evidence. If a CXR is available, shift of the mediastinal structures and tracheal deviation will be evident. If the patient is very unstable and not able to have an erect film taken, a supine may be requested. In this case the costophrenic angles can be seen to be deepened.

(e) In the case of a tension pneumothorax a large cannula (14 gauge) should be inserted through the second intercostal space on the appropriate side. A formal chest drain can then be inserted once the tension is acutely relieved. In the case of a standard pneumothorax, if small and in patients without significant chest disease, it may be allowed to spontaneously resolve, providing daily chest radiographs are taken initially. Others should be treated by simple aspiration or a chest drain (a drain into the intrapleural space).

4. Congestive cardiac failure

(a) This CXR demonstrates cardiomegaly, the heart size being greater than 0.5 of the cardiothoracic ratio on a PA chest radiograph. There is also evidence of upper lobe diversion, seen as increased pulmonary vascular markings.

(b) A transthoracic echocardiogram (echo) would clarify details of cardiac function such as ventricular size, function, degree of impairment and valvular disease. It will also give an estimate of the ejection fraction.

(c) There are five classic features of cardiac failure on CXR: cardiomegaly, upper lobe venous diversion, Kerley B lines, interstitial oedema in the later stages, described classically as 'bat's wings', and pleural effusions.

(d) As the pumping function of the heart becomes impaired, cardiac output is reduced and the heart is unable to 'eject' (pump) all the blood that enters via venous return back into the systemic circulation. This causes back pressure into the venous circulation, resulting in an increase in pulmonary wedge pressure and so diverting blood to the upper lobes. The initial cause of the cardiac malfunction may be an area of dead, and so functionless, myocardium, following a myocardial infarct.

(e) In severe congestive cardiac failure (CCF) the appearance may be confused with acute respiratory distress syndrome (ARDS). Careful attention to heart size will reveal a normal sized heart in ARDS, unlike CCF.

5. Peripheral vascular disease

(a) Images are digital as x-rays are received by an image intensifier, not a traditional x-ray plate, and are stored on a computer as digital images. An initial image is taken of all structures, before contrast is administered. This gives the so-called 'mask' image. A further image is taken with contrast within the vessels. With the use of the computer the mask image is then subtracted (taken away/faded out), leaving a distinct image without visual interference from surrounding structures.

(b) Contrast is seen within the peripheral vascular system at the level of the iliac arteries. There is a tight stenosis of the right iliac artery 3 cm distal to the bifurcation. The subsequent image (Fig. 20.9b) demonstrates restoration of normal vessel calibre following stent placement.

(c) The options are: do nothing, undertake balloon angioplasty, stent the vessel across the stenosis or refer for bypass surgery. A number of factors— including the patient's co-morbidity, location of stenosis/es and number of stenoses—will dictate which management option is chosen.

(d) Positive contrast agents, such as those that are iodine based, absorb x-rays. Consequently fewer x-rays reach the detector or plate and the vessels are seen as areas of radio-opacity. Negative contrast agents, such as carbon dioxide, do not absorb x-rays and so more x-rays reach the detector or plate.

(e) Iodine is the principal component of a positive contrast agent and is filtered and excreted by the kidneys. If a patient has renal impairment the kidneys will be less able to cope with this additional burden and their function may worsen, causing contrast nephropathy. In this case a negative contrast agent may be necessary.

6. Oesophageal carcinoma

(a) There is a stricture in the mid third of the oesophagus with shouldering of the lesion. Luminal diameter is 2 mm at its narrowest.

(b) The patient must be fasted overnight. The patient swallows barium in the erect position and a series of images are taken of the pharynx, oesophagus and stomach.

(c) Strictures which have a shouldered appearance are typically malignant. Intraluminal compression from an eroding tumour mass gives this classic feature.

(d) CT chest and abdomen are undertaken for staging purposes. This will assess mediastinal lymph node enlargement, the extent of the tumour mass, any invasion of surrounding structures and metastatic disease. Where available, endoluminal ultrasound of the oesophagus is valuable in assessing the depth of invasion for those being considered for surgery. There is now also a role for CT–PET in tumour staging.

(e) Oesophageal malignancies are either squamous cell carcinomas or adenocarcinomas. The latter arise in the distal third in metaplastic epithelium from prolonged Barrett's oesophagus which progresses from metaplasia to dysplasia to neoplasia. As both squamous cell carcinomas and adenocarcinomas arise here, it is the commonest location. Location is important as it dictates, in those suitable for surgery, the nature of the procedure: middle third tumours being suitable for an Ivor Lewis procedure whereas distal third have total thoracic oesophagectomy.

7. Pneumoperitoneum

(a) Gas can be seen beneath both hemidiaphragms and is extraluminal, indicating it has entered the peritoneal cavity from a gas-containing structure.

(b) Pneumoperitoneum is seen in any condition causing gas to enter the peritoneal cavity. Examples include: following abdominal surgery, perforated bowel, perforated duodenal ulcer, a biliary leak and gallstone ileus. Postoperatively the gas resolves with time, taking longer in those who are thin—the heavier the patient, the quicker the gas is absorbed.

(c) Various radiological signs have been described, perhaps the two most widely quoted being the 'falciform ligament' sign and 'Rigler's' sign. With Rigler's sign, gas can be seen on both sides (gas within the lumen as expected and gas outside of the bowel in the peritoneal cavity) of the bowel wall, making it look strikingly clear. The falciform ligament extends from the surface of the liver to the umbilicus. Gas within the peritoneal cavity highlights the ligament as gas is on either side of it.

(d) In Chilaiditi's syndrome a loop of bowel is located adjacent to the hemidiaphragm, giving the appearance of a pneumoperitoneum. On closer inspection the luminal markings of the bowel wall can be identified.

(e) The 'double bubble' sign on an erect film is a feature of duodenal atresia. This condition may be congenital or acquired. One bubble represents the normal gastric gas bubble and the other is formed by gas within the duodenum.

8. Large bowel obstruction

(a) This film shows dilated large bowel, 7 cm in diameter. The bowel is located at the periphery of the film and has haustral markings across its lumen.

A 'cut-off point' is seen at the proximal descending colon. There are no faeces or gas distal to this point, implying that the distal bowel is empty.

(b) The diameter of the bowel, markings, location of the bowel on the AXR and number of bowel loops help to confirm whether an obstruction is in the large or small bowel.

(c) Small bowel obstruction can be thought of as a 'picture within a frame' as the bowel loops are in the centre of the film. The commonest cause is from adhesions secondary to previous abdominal surgery.

(d) The 'cut-off sign' is an important radiological sign as it helps to distinguish between mechanical bowel obstruction and pseudo-obstruction or ileus. In mechanical obstruction where a physical blockage exists, such as an intraluminal mass, there is the prevention of the passage of faeces and gas distally. A distinct point will be recognized with time as all the gas/faeces distal to this point are passed PR, leaving an empty bowel.

(e) It may be necessary to investigate further—either immediately or if conservative treatment (drip and suck) is unsuccessful. An instant enema (single contrast) study may be performed to identify obstruction but will not give any mucosal detail. For this, a formal study, after the acute obstruction has resolved, may be appropriate to identify an intraluminal cause for the initial blockage. As an obstructed bowel is at risk of perforation, if this study is undertaken before treatment a water-soluble agent should be used. A CT of the abdomen will often help delineate the cause and confirm the obstruction.

9. Osteoarthritis of the hip

(a, b) The four classic radiological features of OA are: joint space narrowing, osteophyte formation, subchondral sclerosis and bone cyst formation.

(c) Osteophytes are formed as the osteoblasts (cells that lay down bone) attempt to repair damaged areas by laying down new bone.

(d) Osteoarthritis may be primary or secondary. Primary osteoarthritis is characterized by primary nodal disease that typically occurs in postmenopausal women with associated hand features of Heberden's and/or Bouchard's nodes. The causes can be remembered easily as they all start with the letter 'I': Idiopathic, Ischaemic, Incongruency, Injury, Inflammation and Interesting others (e.g. acromegaly).

10. Breast carcinoma

(a) As with the general principle of imaging, orthogonal views are taken—two views at right angles to each other. A single plain film may not give an accurate assessment of a three-dimensional structure. Therefore two views of the breast are routinely taken—a craniocaudal (head to toe) and an oblique.

(b) There is an irregular mass in the left breast. It is spiculated in nature and contains areas of microcalcification. This is most likely a breast carcinoma.

(c) Given that the diagnosis is most likely breast carcinoma, a tissue diagnosis is needed by FNAC or core biopsy, often under ultrasound guidance and on occasion by stereotactic biopsy which would be performed by the radiologist. When a confirmed diagnosis of carcinoma is made, staging of the tumour is indicated—this would include a CT of the chest and abdomen given breast carcinoma's preponderance to metastasize to the lungs and liver.

(d) Mammography utilizes x-rays to visualize the breast parenchyma. The clarity of distinguishing a breast lump from normal tissue is therefore dependent on differences in tissue density. The breast is composed of chiefly glandular and adipose tissue. In the young premenopausal breast the proportion of glandular tissue is high. This is similar in density to a tumour mass and thus identification can be difficult. As the breast ages, the proportion of adipose to glandular tissue increases. Mammography then becomes more useful. In the under 35 year olds ultrasound is the imaging modality of choice, or at least as a supplement to mammography.

(e) Due to both the greater ability to treat breast cancer and cosmetic enhancement by breast augmentation, patients presenting for imaging with breast prostheses are quite common. The prosthesis may make visualization of the breast and any suspected lump difficult by standard screening views. Therefore further projections may be necessary or imaging with MRI.

Glossary

AAA	abdominal aortic aneurysm		DTPA	diethylene triamine pentacetic acid
ABG	arterial blood gas		DVT	deep venous thrombosis
ABPI	ankle brachial pressure index		ECA	external carotid artery
AC	abdominal circumference		ECG	electrocardiogram
AF	atrial fibrillation		ED	effective dose
ANA	antinuclear antibody		EDH	extradural haematoma
AP	anteroposterior		ERCP	endoscopic retrograde cholangiopancreatography
APKD	adult polycystic kidney disease		ESM	ejection systolic murmur
APN	acute pyelonephritis		ESR	erythrocyte sedimentation rate
ARDS	acute respiratory distress syndrome		EVAR	endovascular repair [of abdominal aortic aneurysms]
ASD	atrial septal defect			
AV	atrioventricular		FBP	full blood picture
AVM	arteriovenous malformation		FDG	fluorodeoxyglucose
AVN	avascular necrosis		FEV_1	forced expiratory volume in 1 sec
AVSD	atrioventricular septal defect		FL	femur length
AXR	abdominal X-ray		FNAC	fine needle aspiration cytology
BMI	body mass index		FNH	focal nodular hyperplasia
BPD	biparietal diameter		FVC	forced vital capacity
CABG	coronary artery bypass graft		GCS	Glasgow Coma Scale
CAM	cystic adenomatoid malformation		GI	gastrointestinal
CBD	common bile duct		GORD	gastro-oesophageal reflux disease
CC	corpus callosum		Hb	haemoglobin
CCF	congestive cardiac failure		HC	head circumference
CEA	carcinoembryonic antigen		HCC	hepatocellular carcinoma
CF	cystic fibrosis		HCG	human chorionic gonadotrophin
COPD	chronic obstructive pulmonary disease		HIDA	hepatoiminodiacetic acid
CPPD	calcium pyrophosphate deposition disease		HOCM	hypertrophic obstructive cardiomyopathy
CRC	colorectal carcinoma		HPOA	hypertrophic pulmonary osteoarthropathy
CRL	crown–rump length			
CRP	C-reactive protein		HRCT	high resolution computed tomography
CSF	cerebrospinal fluid		HS	heart sound(s)
CSP	cavum septum pellucidum		IBD	inflammatory bowel disease
CT	computed tomography		ICA	internal carotid artery
CTA	CT angiography		ICH	intracerebral haematoma; intracranial haemorrhage
CVA	cerebrovascular accident			
CXR	chest X-ray		ICP	intracranial pressure
DAI	diffuse axonal injury		ICU	intensive care unit
DCBE	double contrast barium enema		IIH	idiopathic intracranial hypertension
DDH	developmental dysplasia of the hip		INR	international normalized ratio
DEXA	dual energy X-ray absorptiometry		IR	inversion recovery
DIP	distal interphalangeal [joint]		IRMER	Ionizing Radiation Medical Exposure Regulations
DMARD	disease-modifying anti-rheumatic drug			
DMSA	dimercaptosuccinic acid		IUGR	intrauterine growth retardation
DSA	digital subtraction angiography			

IVC	inferior vena cava	PEFR	peak expiratory flow rate
IVH	intraventricular haemorrhage	PET	positron emission tomography
IVU	intravenous urogram	PFT	pulmonary function test
JVP	jugular venous pressure	PIP	proximal interphalangeal [joint]
LA	left atrium	PPI	proton pump inhibitor
LFT	liver function test	PR	per rectum
LIF	left iliac fossa	PTC	percutaneous transhepatic
LMP	last menstrual period		cholangiography
LMWH	low molecular weight heparin	RA	rheumatoid arthritis; right atrium
LV	left ventricle	RBBB	right bundle branch block
LVF	left ventricular failure	RF	radiofrequency; rheumatoid factor
MAA	macroaggregates of albumin	RI	resistive index
MAG-3	mercaptoacetyltriglycene	RIP	rotation, inspiration, penetration
MCP	metacarpophalangeal [joint]	RTA	road traffic accident
MCUG	micturating cystourethrography	RUQ	right upper quadrant
MCV	mean corpuscular volume	RV	right ventricle
MDP	methylene diphosphonate	SAH	subarachnoid haemorrhage
MIBG	meta-iodo-benzyl-guanidine	SB	spina bifida
MIBI	methoxyisobutyl isonitrile	SCFE	slipped capital femoral epiphysis
MRA	magnetic resonance angiography	SDH	subdural haematoma
MRC	magnetic resonance cholangiography	SLE	systemic lupus erythematosus
MRCP	magnetic resonance	SMA	superior mesenteric artery
	cholangiopancreatography	SOB	shortness of breath
MRI	magnetic resonance imaging	SPECT	single photon emission computed
MSAFP	maternal serum alphafetoprotein		tomography
NAD	no abnormal defect	STIR	short tau inversion-recovery
NAI	non-accidental injury	SUFE	slipped upper femoral epiphysis
NCCT	non-contrast computed tomography	TAS	transabdominal scan
NEC	necrotizing enterocolitis	TB	tuberculosis
NG	nasogastric [tube]	TFT	thyroid function test
NM	nuclear medicine	THR	total hip replacement
NSAID	non-steroidal anti-inflammatory drug	TIA	transient ischaemic attack
NT	nuchal translucency	TOE	transoesophageal echocardiography
NTD	neural tube defects	TTE	transthoracic echocardiography
OA	osteoarthritis	TVUS	transvaginal ultrasound scan
OCP	oral contraceptive pill	U&E	urea and electrolytes
PA	posteroanterior	UC	ulcerative colitis
PAPVD	partial anomalous pulmonary venous	USS	ultrasound scan
	drainage	UTI	urinary tract infection
PCA	percutaneous coronary angioplasty	VQ scan	ventilation–perfusion scan
PCom	posterior communicating [artery]	VSD	ventricular septal defect
PDA	patent ductus arteriosus	VUR	vesico-ureteric reflux
PE	pulmonary embolus	WCC	white cell count

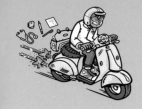

Index